INTERVENTIONAL CARDIOLOGY CLINICS

www.interventional.theclinics.com

Editor-in-Chief

MARVIN H. ENG

Tricuspid Valve Interventions

January 2022 • Volume 11 • Number 1

Editors

VASILIS C. BABALIAROS

ADAM B. GREENBAUM

ELSEVIER

1600 John F. Kennedy Boulevard • Suite 1800 • Philadelphia, Pennsylvania, 19103-2899

http://www.theclinics.com

INTERVENTIONAL CARDIOLOGY CLINICS Volume 11, Number 1
January 2022 ISSN 2211-7458, ISBN-13: 978-0-323-89696-2

Editor: Joanna Collett
Developmental Editor: Arlene B. Campos

Interventional Cardiology Clinics (ISSN 2211-7458) is published quarterly by Elsevier Inc., 360 Park Avenue South, New York, NY 10010-1710. Months of issue are January, April, July, and October. Subscription prices are USD 209 per year for US individuals, USD 641 for US institutions, USD 100 per year for US students, USD 209 per year for Canadian individuals, USD 660 for Canadian institutions, USD 100 per year for Canadian students, USD 296 per year for international individuals, USD 660 for international institutions, and USD 150 per year for international students. To receive student/resident rate, orders must be accompanied by name of affiliated institution, date of term, and the *signature* of program/residency coordinator on institution letterhead. Orders will be billed at individual rate until proof of status is received. Foreign air speed delivery is included in all *Clinics* subscription prices. All prices are subject to change without notice. **POSTMASTER:** Send address changes to *Interventional Cardiology Clinics*, Elsevier Health Sciences Division, Subscription Customer Service, 3251 Riverport Lane, Maryland Heights, MO 63043. **Customer Service: Telephone: 1-800-654-2452** (U.S. and Canada); **1-314-447-8871** (outside U.S. and Canada). **Fax: 1-314-447-8029.** E-mail: journalscustomerservice-usa@elsevier.com (for print support); journalsonlinesupport-usa@elsevier.com (for online support).

Reprints. For copies of 100 or more of articles in this publication, please contact the Commercial Reprints Department, Elsevier Inc., 360 Park Avenue South, New York, NY 10010-1710. Tel.: 212-633-3874; Fax: 212-633-3820; E-mail: reprints@elsevier.com.

CONTRIBUTORS

EDITOR-IN-CHIEF

MARVIN H. ENG, MD
Structural Heart Program Medical Director,
Structural Heart Disease Fellowship Director,
Director of Cardiovascular Quality, Banner
University Medical Center, Phoenix, Arizona,
USA

EDITORS

VASILIS C. BABALIAROS, MD
Co-Director, Structural Heart and Valve
Center, Department of Internal
Medicine-Cardiology, Emory University,
Atlanta, Georgia, USA

ADAM B. GREENBAUM, MD
Co-Director, Structural Heart and Valve
Center, Department of Internal Medicine–
Cardiology, Emory University, Atlanta,
Georgia, USA

AUTHORS

ISLAM ABUDAYYEH, MD
Division of Cardiology, Loma Linda University,
Loma Linda, California, USA

FAEEZ M. ALI, MD
Division of Cardiology, St. Michael's Hospital,
Toronto, Ontario, Canada; Waikato Hospital,
Hamilton, New Zealand

MOHAMMAD REZA AMINI, MD
Division of Cardiology, Loma Linda University,
Loma Linda, California, USA

VASILIS C. BABALIAROS, MD
Co-Director, Structural Heart and Valve
Center, Department of Internal Medicine-
Cardiology, Emory University, Atlanta,
Georgia, USA

VINAYAK N. BAPAT, MBBS
Valve Science Center, Minneapolis Heart
Institute Foundation, Minneapolis Heart
Institute, Abbott Northwestern Hospital,
Minneapolis, Minnesota, USA

SHARON BRUOHA, MD
Department of Cardiology, Montefiore
Medical Center, Bronx, New York, USA

JOÃO L. CAVALCANTE, MD
Valve Science Center, Minneapolis Heart
Institute Foundation, Minneapolis Heart

Institute, Abbott Northwestern Hospital,
Minneapolis, Minnesota, USA; Director,
Cardiovascular Imaging Research Center and
Core Laboratory

MEI CHAU, MD
Department of Cardiology, Montefiore
Medical Center, Bronx, New York, USA

HENRYK DREGER, MD
Charité–University Hospital Berlin, Berlin,
Germany

MARVIN H. ENG, MD
Structural Heart Program Medical Director,
Structural Heart Disease Fellowship Director,
Director of Cardiovascular Quality, Banner
University Medical Center, Phoenix, Arizona,
USA

NEIL P. FAM, MD, MSc
Division of Cardiology, St. Michael's Hospital,
Toronto, Ontario, Canada

KENITH FANG, MD
Chief of Cardiothoracic Surgery, Banner
University Medical Center, Phoenix, Arizona,
USA

HANS R. FIGULLA, MD
University Heart Center, Jena, Germany

PATRICK T. GLEASON, MD
Division of Cardiology, Emory University
Hospital, Division of Cardiology, Emory
Structural Heart and Valve Center, Atlanta,
Georgia, USA

YTHAN GOLDBERG, MD
Department of Cardiology, Montefiore
Medical Center, Bronx, New York, USA

ADAM B. GREENBAUM, MD
Co-Director, Structural Heart and Valve
Center, Department of Internal
Medicine-Cardiology, Emory University,
Atlanta, Georgia, USA

DANIEL HAGEMEYER, MD
Division of Cardiology, St. Michael's Hospital,
Toronto, Ontario, Canada

MICHAEL E. HALKOS, MD, MSc
Professor of Surgery, Chief, Division of
Cardiothoracic Surgery, Department of
Surgery, Emory University School of Medicine,
Atlanta, Georgia, USA

GO HASHIMOTO, MD
Cardiovascular Imaging Research Center and
Core Lab, Minneapolis Heart Institute
Foundation, Minneapolis, Minnesota, USA

EDWIN C. HO, MD
Department of Cardiology, Montefiore
Medical Center, Bronx, New York, USA

AMALIA A. JONSSON, MD
Assistant Professor of Surgery, Division of
Cardiothoracic Surgery, Department of
Surgery, Emory University School of Medicine,
Atlanta, Georgia, USA

AZEEM LATIB, MD
Department of Cardiology, Montefiore
Medical Center, Bronx, New York, USA

MICHAEL LAULE, MD
Charité–University Hospital Berlin, Berlin,
Germany

ALEXANDER LAUTEN, MD
Helios Klinikum Erfurt GmbH, Erfurt,
Thuringia, Germany; Department of
Cardiology, Helios Clinic Erfurt, Germany

BERNARDO B.C. LOPES, MD
Cardiovascular Imaging Research Center and
Core Lab, Minneapolis Heart Institute
Foundation, Minneapolis, Minnesota, USA

ANTONIO MANGIERI, MD
Department of Invasive Cardiology,
Humanitas Clinical and Research Center,
IRCCS, Milan, Italy

GEORG NICKENIG, MD
Professor, Heart Centre, Department of
Cardiology, University Hospital Bonn, Bonn,
Germany

GERALDINE ONG, MD, MSc
Division of Cardiology, St. Michael's Hospital,
Toronto, Ontario, Canada

PRAPAIPAN PUTTHAPIBAN, MD
Division of Cardiology, Loma Linda University,
Loma Linda, California, USA

PRADHUM RAM, MD
Division of Cardiology, Emory University
Hospital, Atlanta, Georgia, USA

MARKUS D. SCHERER, MD
Sanger Heart & Vascular Institute Adult
Cardiology Kenilworth, Charlotte, North
Carolina, USA

NIKOLOZ SHEKILADZE, MD
Division of Cardiology, Emory University
Hospital, Atlanta, Georgia, USA

PAUL SORAJJA, MD
Valve Science Center, Minneapolis Heart
Institute Foundation, Minneapolis Heart
Institute, Abbott Northwestern Hospital,
Minneapolis, Minnesota, USA

KARL STANGL, MD
Charité–University Hospital Berlin, Berlin,
Germany

VINOD THOURANI, MD
Marcus Chief of Cardiovascular Surgery,
Piedmont Heart Institute, Atlanta, Georgia,
USA

JOHANNA VOGELHUBER, MD
Heart Centre, Department of Cardiology,
University Hospital Bonn, Bonn, Germany

MARCEL WEBER, MD
Heart Centre, Department of Cardiology,
University Hospital Bonn, Bonn, Germany

JOE XIE, MD
Division of Cardiology, Emory University
Hospital, Division of Cardiology, Emory

Structural Heart and Valve Center, Atlanta,
Georgia, USA

PRADEEP YADAV, MD
Division of Cardiology, Piedmont Heart
Institute, Atlanta, Georgia, USA

CONTENTS

Transcatheter valve interventions have seen a significant increase in the past decade. The combination of improved techniques and available tools provides less invasive options supplementing surgical therapies. The tricuspid valve (TV) apparatus is a complex structure between the right atrium and the right ventricle; it generally consists of 3 leaflets (anterior, posterior, and septal) inserted in the fibrous tricuspid annulus and connected to the papillary muscle via the chordae tendinae. This article reviews TV anatomy, the pathophysiology of tricuspid regurgitation, and multimodality imaging to study TV, as well as provides an overview of transcatheter TV intervention.

 Video content accompanies this article at http://www.interventional.theclinics.com

Transcatheter tricuspid valve (TV) interventions have increased dramatically in recent years. TV imaging is challenging in many respects. Given the TV's anatomic complexity, multimodality imaging, which is centered on echocardiography (echo), plays a significant part in planning and execution of these interventions. With the help of echo-guided imaging, pathophysiologic mechanisms for TV disease are better understood, and thus, appropriate valve intervention can be strategized. Novel devices for the TV continue to be developed, and thus, intraprocedural echo imaging will continue to evolve in the days ahead.

 Video content accompanies this article at http://www.interventional.theclinics.com.

Transcatheter tricuspid valve interventions (TTVIs) are rapidly growing as a less invasive treatment of high surgical risk patients with advanced TR. A comprehensive anatomic and functional assessment of the tricuspid valve and right-sided chambers is essential for candidate selection and procedural planning. Advanced imaging with cardiac computed tomography (CCT) and cardiac magnetic resonance (CMR) can provide accurate anatomic and functional assessment of the tricuspid valve, its apparatus, and the right-sided chambers. In this review, we provide an updated overview of the emerging role of CCT and CMR for TR patient evaluation, TTVI planning, and follow-up.

Severe tricuspid regurgitation renders patients frail, and surgical treatment is associated with high mortality. Because most of the tricuspid regurgitation patients are functional and have significant annular dilation, large coaptation gaps are seen. This anatomy is best addressed with transcatheter tricuspid valve replacement (TTVR), and promising therapies are under clinical investigation. Most TTVR devices are in early clinical development with one transcatheter heart valve in pivotal trial; TTVR is expected to significantly affect tricuspid regurgitation and survival.

Transcathetertherapy has expanded the treatment options for patients with heart valve disease. Interventional therapy for aortic, mitral, and pulmonic valve disease is well established; however, catheter-based approaches to tricuspid regurgitation (TR) are still in early stages of development. For some of the interventional concepts to TR, including the edge-to-edge-repair, transcatheter annuloplasty, the tricuspid spacer, and caval valves, procedural feasibility and favorable early clinical outcome have been demonstrated in small compassionate case series. This article reviews the pathophysiological background and current evidence for caval valve implantation and examines the potential role of this approach for the treatment of severe TR.

The prevalence of severe tricuspid regurgitation in older patients is high, and the clinical relevance is perceived more and more in recent years. Many of these patients are not suitable for surgery because of their age and comorbidities. Therefore, a variety of percutaneous interventions have been developed to address this unmet need. Procedural success strongly depends on adequate imaging during the intervention. Although transesophageal echocardiography is the standard of care, imaging may be limited due to anatomic factors and adverse acoustic shadowing. In this review, we discuss the current and future role of intracardiac echocardiography in tricuspid valve interventions.

TRICUSPID VALVE INTERVENTIONS

RELATED SERIES

Cardiology Clinics
https://www.cardiology.theclinics.com/
Heart Failure Clinics
https://www.heartfailure.theclinics.com/
Cardiac Electrophysiology Clinics
https://www.cardiacep.theclinics.com/

THE CLINICS ARE NOW AVAILABLE ONLINE!

Access your subscription at:
www.theclinics.com

FOREWORD

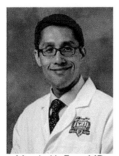

Marvin H. Eng, MD
Consulting Editor

We are pleased to introduce this issue of *Interventional Cardiology Clinics* that discusses the state-of-the-art in tricuspid valve interventions. As tricuspid regurgitation was once considered a bystander lesion, improved appreciation for the prognostic significance of tricuspid regurgitation has made it a focus for investigational therapies.

Tricuspid regurgitation is uniquely challenging for percutaneous intervention due to the low-flow hemodynamic milieu and relatively thin supporting structures for anchoring devices. Identical to other transcatheter innovations, the tools for treatment revolve around anatomy. Tricuspid anatomy was underappreciated, and fresh perspective from pathologic and imaging studies now has improved the feasibility of repair and replacement. Multimodality imaging from both echocardiography and computed tomography is essential for screening and procedural planning, similar to other structural procedures. Like mitral therapies, intraprocedural echocardiography plays a major role, but, in addition to transesophageal, intracardiac echocardiography can be a useful

and sometimes necessary adjunct. Edge-to-edge repair, percutaneous annuloplasty, orthotopic valve replacement, and heterotopic valve implantation are thus far the main contenders for tricuspid therapies, and all are explored in this issue.

This issue of *Interventional Cardiology Clinics* has been edited by Drs Greenbaum and Babaliaros, both experts in structural heart interventions and innovation. They have assembled a compendium of articles to guide us on the path toward understanding contemporary and future therapies for severe tricuspid valve regurgitation.

Marvin H. Eng, MD
Banner University Medical Center
1111 East McDowell Road
Phoenix, AZ 85006, USA

E-mail address:
engm@email.arizona.edu

Intervent Cardiol Clin 11 (2022) xi
https://doi.org/10.1016/j.iccl.2021.11.001
2211-7458/22/© 2021 Published by Elsevier Inc.

PREFACE

The Final Frontier in Valvular Heart Therapies: Tricuspid Regurgitation

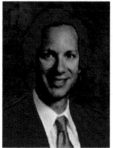 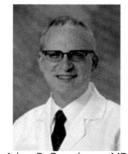

Vasilis C. Babaliaros, MD   Adam B. Greenbaum, MD
Editors

Fresh appreciation for the tricuspid pathologic condition and its prognostic implications has ushered in a burst of interest for treating tricuspid regurgitation. As tricuspid regurgitation is often a secondary lesion to mitral valve disease or cardiomyopathy, therapies were directed to the primary disease. However, treatment of primary lesions (eg, mitral disease, cardiomyopathy) may not resolve tricuspid regurgitation, and residual valvular incompetence negatively impacts survival. Therefore, considerable enthusiasm is currently directed at innovating viable solutions. Careful anatomic study from both pathologic and imaging perspectives is key to screening, selecting, and planning interventions. We have provided an article for pathologic anatomic study, echocardiography, and computed tomography to illustrate the subtle complexities of the tricuspid apparatus. Detailed foreknowledge is necessary for successful intervention, and the leaps in imaging for tricuspid valve are reviewed by noninvasive thought leaders. The predicate for percutaneous treatment is surgery; thus, an in-depth look at surgical repair and replacement techniques is provided in this compendium. Even surgical treatment of tricuspid regurgitation has limited durability, and the specific nuances to treating failed bioprostheses and repairs are discussed at length.

Although surgical repair is the standard that percutaneous procedures hope to meet, edge-to-edge repair and annuloplasty are current techniques being utilized and under investigation at this time. As the nature of most tricuspid regurgitation is valvular incompetence caused by annular dilation, sometimes the valvular coaptation gap renders most contemporary repair techniques ineffective. Consequently, investigators have devoted efforts to develop orthotopic valve replacement, an area of intense development. Still in its initial stages, orthotopic valve replacement does provide an attractive solution to abolishing tricuspid regurgitation but is accompanied by the prerequisite for anticoagulation. Finally, for patients without anatomy compatible with current therapies, heterotopic valve implantation has been an unconventional solution to protect visceral organs from elevated right-sided pressures by placing bioprostheses in the superior and inferior vena cava. Intuitively, this may appear to be a timely solution, but the reported results are mixed, and we await confirmatory data of its efficacy. All in all, this issue of *Interventional Cardiology Clinics* provides a detailed summary of the contemporary advances in tricuspid valve therapy. We are grateful for the expert and thorough

Intervent Cardiol Clin 11 (2022) xiii–xiv
https://doi.org/10.1016/j.iccl.2021.11.002
2211-7458/22/© 2021 Published by Elsevier Inc.

review by several luminary interventional cardiologists within this text.

Vasilis C. Babaliaros, MD
Structural Heart and Valve Center
Department of Internal Medicine–Cardiology
Emory University
550 Peachtree St Ne
Medical, Office Tower, Fl 6
Atlanta, GA 30308, USA

Adam B. Greenbaum, MD
Structural Heart and Valve Center
Department of Internal Medicine–Cardiology
Emory University
550 Peachtree St Ne
Medical, Office Tower, Fl 6
Atlanta, GA 30308, USA

E-mail addresses:
vbabali@emory.edu (V.C. Babaliaros)
Adam.b.greenbaum@emory.edu (A.B. Greenbaum)

Anatomy of the Tricuspid Valve and Pathophysiology of Tricuspid Regurgitation

Prapaipan Putthapiban, MD,
Mohammad Reza Amini, MD, Islam Abudayyeh, MD*

KEYWORDS

• Tricuspid valve • Right ventricle • Anatomy • Tricuspid regurgitation

---

KEY POINTS

- The tricuspid valve is an anatomically variable valve with direct effect on right heart loading.
- Transcatheter options for addressing tricuspid valve dysfunction are limited but developing. This is due to the variability and surrounding anatomy.
- Understanding the location of the valve relative to the right ventricle, outflow, inferior, and superior vena cavas is essential for safe intervention.

Transcatheter valve interventions have seen a significant increase in the past decade. The combination of improved techniques and available tools provides less invasive options supplementing surgical therapies.[1] The initial focus for such interventions had been primarily the aortic valve, but recently more attention is being paid to the mitral, pulmonic, and tricuspid valves. Although early in development, several devices are currently in preclinical development or trials. Hemodynamically, the tricuspid valve operates at a lower pressure than the left-sided heart valves; however, it enables insidious development of volume overload and pathologic remodeling to cause significant damage to the heart.

The tricuspid valve (TV) apparatus is a complex structure between the right atrium (RA) and the right ventricle (RV); it generally consists of 3 leaflets (anterior, posterior, and septal) inserted in the fibrous tricuspid annulus (TA) and connected to the papillary muscle via the chordae tendinae. The TV apparatus is often referred to as the "forgotten valve" due to the initial assessment of its role as a bystander that improved with concomitant mitral valve disease was adequately treated.[2] The dysfunctions of TV are primarily consequences of left-sided valvular disease or myocardial disease. Tricuspid regurgitation (TR) is common, affecting 65% to 85% of adults.[3,4] The prevalence of hemodynamically significant TR is about 1.6 million persons in the United States.[5] Moreover, moderate to severe TR is associated with increased mortality independent of pulmonary pressure and RV dysfunction.[6] At present, American and European guidelines recommend TV intervention (repair or replace) at the time of left-sided valve surgery in severe TR (class I) or TA dilation regardless of TR severity (class IIa). In symptomatic severe primary TR or asymptomatic primary TR with progressive RV dysfunction, TV intervention is recommended as a standalone procedure with the caveat of weak evidence base for efficacy (class IIb).[7,8] In high-surgical-risk patients, transcatheter procedures for the TV can potentially be an alternative option. Owing to the 3-dimensional (3D) complexity of the surrounding anatomy, the pathophysiology of TR, multimodality imaging, as well as the valve itself, a thorough understanding of the anatomy is fundamental to selecting the approach and safely performing such procedures. This article reviews TV anatomy, the pathophysiology of TR, and multimodality imaging to study TV, as well as provides an overview of transcatheter TV intervention.

Division of Cardiology, Loma Linda University, 2068 Orange Tree Lane, Suite 215, Loma Linda, CA 92374, USA
* Corresponding author. 11234 Anderson Street, Loma Linda, CA 92354.
E-mail address: iabudayyeh@mac.com

Intervent Cardiol Clin 11 (2022) 1–9
https://doi.org/10.1016/j.iccl.2021.09.003
2211-7458/22/© 2021 Elsevier Inc. All rights reserved.

ANATOMY OF THE TRICUSPID VALVE

The TV is the atrioventricular (AV) valve located between the RA and the RV. TV is the most apically positioned and the largest valve with an average orifice diameter of 20 mm/m^2 and an area of 5.8 cm^2/m^2.[9] There are 4 components of TV: the leaflets, the papillary muscles, the chordae tendinae, and the TA. The normal valvular function depends on both valvular components and adjacent RA and RV. The TV complex and adjacent structures are illustrated in Figs. 1 and 2.

Tricuspid Valve Leaflets

TV is truly trileaflet in only 57% of the healthy subjects; bicuspid and more than 3 leaflets may be present as normal variants.[10] The 3 TV leaflets are named according to their anatomic position: anterior, septal, and posterior leaflet.[11] The anterior leaflet is the largest, with a quadrangular shape covering the major part of the orifice and the greatest motion. The posterior leaflet is the shortest with multiple scallops. There may not be a clear separation from the anterior leaflet in approximately 10% of the population.[12] The septal leaflet is the least mobile leaflet with a semicircular shape. Compared with the insertion of the anterior mitral leaflet, the septal leaflet of TV is inserted at less than or equal to 10 mm closer to the apex (Fig. 3). Anatomic landmarks of the leaflets are varied, except the commissure between septal and posterior leaflets is normally located near the entrance of the coronary sinus (CS) into the RA. A comparison of the leaflets of TV with mitral valve shows that the TV leaflets are very thin and relatively fragile. Leaflet calcification is rarely seen. The coaptation length of the TV is about 5 to 10 mm, which is usually located at the TA level.

Subvalvular Apparatus

There are a variable number of papillary muscles in the RV.[12,13] The anterior papillary muscle is the largest papillary muscle that arises from RV free wall and trabecular septomarginalis (see Fig. 3). This muscle lends chordal support to the anterior and posterior leaflet. The posterior papillary muscle, often bifid or trifid, arises from the posterior aspect of RV with its chordae connecting posterior and septal leaflets. The septal papillary muscle can be least prominent or even absent in up to 20% of the normal population.[14] The chordae can arise directly from the septum to the anterior and septal leaflets. Dilation of the RV or displacement of the papillary muscle will affect tricuspid leaflet coaptation due to the fixed length of the chordae. Unlike mitral valve tensor apparatus, chordae of TV are more fragile and may interfere with catheters or more easily be damaged during transcatheter interventions such as lead insertions and biopsies.

Tricuspid Annulus

The TA is a nonplanar saddle shape with a larger curved segment at the free wall of the RA and the RV and a shorter straight segment at the septal, which is fairly fixed. The anteroseptal and posterolateral portions are the higher points, whereas the anterolateral and posteroseptal parts are the lower points.[15] TA is very dynamic throughout the cardiac cycle. There is an approximately 30% reduction in the annular area during systole compared with diastole.[16] The geometry of TA can be distorted due to dilation of the RA, RV, or aortic root. In patients with functional TR, the TA became more planar and circular from primary dilation in the RV free wall (anterior) direction as shown in Fig. 1.[17]

There are several essential structures adjacent to TA. First, the right coronary artery (RCA), which normally arises from the right CS, courses down the right AV groove close to the anterior and posterior aspect of the TA. The course of the RCA can be as close as 2 mm in 7% to 8% of patients, which increases the risk of compression or damage during TA intervention.[8] Second, the AV node is located superior to the anteroseptal part of the TA. The triangle of Koch has been used as the anatomic landmark of the AV node; it consists of the tendon of Todaro, which lies above the eustachian valve (posterior border), CS ostium (anterior border), and AV node (medial border) (Fig. 4). AV node continues caudally to His bundle, which runs underneath the membranous septum, posterior

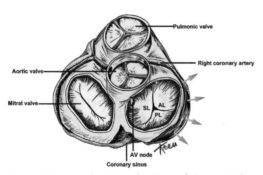

Fig. 1. Diagram depicting the base of the ventricles, after removal of the atria. The RCA courses down the right AV groove close to the anterior and posterior aspect of the TA. The blue arrows demonstrate the direction of TA dilation. AL, anterior leaflet; PL, posterior leaflet; RCA, right coronary artery; SL, septal leaflet.

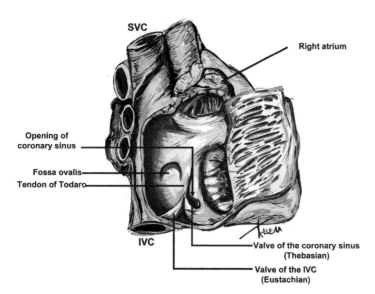

Fig. 2. Diagram depicting the tricuspid valve from the atrial side. The important anatomic landmark for AV node is the triangle of Koch; it consists of the tendon of Todaro, which lies above the eustachian valves (posterior border), coronary sinus ostium (anterior border), and AV node (medial border). SVC, superior vena, cava; IVC, inferior vena cava.

to the anteroseptal commissure.[18] Compression or damage to the AV node or bundle of His can cause a complete AV block that may require permanent pacemaker implantation.[19] Third, the non-CS of Valsalva is located next to the commissure between the anterior and septal leaflets, and the septum there is named the retroaortic rim. Aortic perforation is one of the possible complications of transcatheter intervention of the TV especially because more robust devices are introduced via the inferior vena cava (IVC), which points toward the fossa ovalis and the intraatrial septum just above the TV. Last, the atrial-caval tricuspid isthmus is highly variable across patients and may include a prominent eustachian ridge or Chiari networks that can impact catheter manipulation or device delivery.[20,21]

The anterior leaflet is sometimes redundant and tethered resulting in significant TR. An important consideration during transcatheter interventions is that, unlike the mitral valve relationship to the aortic valve and left ventricular outflow, the TV is not directly adjacent to the RV outflow and there is not a continuity between it and the pulmonic valve. Furthermore, the trabeculations of the RV can interact with bulky devices and large-curve wires in the RV limiting the freedom of movement once caught up in the structures.

PATHOPHYSIOLOGY OF TRICUSPID REGURGITATION

The degree of TR is variable depending on fluid and volume status. TR is common and can be

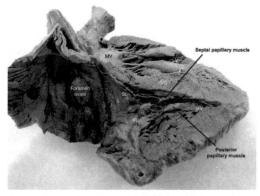

Fig. 3. Tricuspid valve and right ventricle anatomy. The figure displays an anatomic specimen of the TV apparatus and the relationship of the TV to the MV. MV, mitral valve; LV, left ventricle; IVS, interventricular septum.

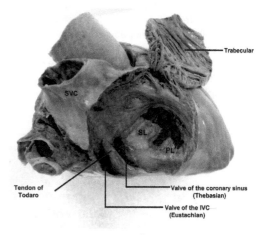

Fig. 4. Tricuspid valve and right atrium anatomy. The figure displays an anatomic specimen with a view of the tricuspid valve from the right atrium.

classified into primary (organic) TR and secondary (functional) TR. More than 90% of TR is secondary TR caused by progressive annular dilation from left-sided heart disease, pulmonary hypertension (PH), RV dysfunction, or atrial fibrillation.[16,22] Primary TR accounts for less than 10% of all TR.[23,24] The causes of primary TR include infective endocarditis, carcinoid, rheumatic heart disease, radiation, RV biopsy, interference from implanted devices such as pacemaker leads, genetic connective tissue disorder, or congenital malformation.[25–27] Whichever cause of TR is present, it usually causes a vicious cycle of worsening TR by increasing annular dilation, RV dilation, and dysfunction.[28]

A significant factor in developing TV regurgitation is PH. PH can bring about RV dilation, annular dilation, and valvular regurgitation. The TV leaflets do not accommodate significant increases in pressure unlike left-sided valves and subsequently leak. Chronically elevated pulmonary pressures may eventually cause the RV to fail, resulting in low right-sided pressure, sometimes described as a "burned out" RV. Conversely, high gradients measured by echocardiography can be a consequence of multiple factors such as shunting or elevated right-sided blood volumes. Therefore, to ascertain a complete picture before an intervention, imaging, hemodynamics and physiology, as well as assessment of cardiac pathological remodeling should all be taken into account.[29]

The TV is quite large giving it the largest diameter of any valve in the heart. The right side of the heart has much lower pressures while having greater volume. As a trileaflet valve, the opening is also the largest; this provides minimal gradient across this anatomy and allows unimpeded flow from the RA into the RV. Owing to the low-pressure nature of the right side of the heart, even minimal obstruction of the valve may cause significant effects on the RA, superior vena cava (SVC), and IVC causing hepatic, abdominal, and peripheral congestion; this can be quite pronounced inducing liver injury and gut edema. Some disease processes such as protein-losing enteropathy have been implicated in elevated right-sided venous pressures and gut edema. Hepatic injury and protein-losing enteropathy render patients with severe TR fragile, intolerant to the extremes of hemodynamic stress, and at times, coagulopathic from coagulation factor deficiencies.

IMAGING FOR TRANSCATHETER INTERVENTIONS IN TRICUSPID VALVE DISEASE

Cardiac imaging has the following crucial roles in transcatheter intervention in TV disease: (1) preprocedural planning including diagnosis, cause, TR severity and RV size and function; (2) procedural guidance; and (3) postprocedural follow-up. Both transthoracic echocardiography (TTE) and transesophageal echocardiography (TEE) are cornerstones for imaging evaluation. TTE usually provides good imaging because TV is located anteriorly. Two-dimensional (2D) echocardiographic imaging rarely offers visualization of 3 TV leaflets simultaneously. It is challenging to predict the combination of TV leaflets seen in any of the standard 2D views.[30] In standard RV inflow view, the anterior leaflet is always seen, whereas in apical 4-chamber view, the septal leaflet is consistently presented.[31] There are adjacent structure landmarks for TV leaflet identification. CS, LV outflow tract, and aortic valve are associated with posterior leaflet, septal leaflet, and anterior leaflet, respectively. 3D echocardiographic imaging provides an accurate leaflet identification of TV; however, it is operator and image quality dependent, as well as limited by anatomy such as left atrial size or shadowing from left-sided structures (Fig. 5). Further investigation with TEE is usually helpful, especially intraoperative. TV can be seen in at least 8 of the 28 standard views in the recent American Society of Echocardiography guidelines for performing a comprehensive intraoperative TEE[32] (Fig. 6). As the RV and the TV are oriented anterior in the heart and further from the esophagus, TEE imaging is much more limited for this valve compared with the mitral and aortic valves; this will present challenges when perfuming echo-guided procedures such as TV clip.

Another imaging approach is the use of intracardiac echocardiography (ICE) (Fig.7). The imaging probe is introduced via the femoral vein most often and advanced to the home position in the RA. From this position, the operator will first see the RA at the top, the RV at the bottom, and the TV between them. Rotating the probe clockwise and counterclockwise will bring into view the different leaflets going from anterior to septal leaflet with clockwise rotation. Right and left angulation of the probe will bring into view different aspects of the valve. With careful flexion, manipulation, and gently advancing the probe the operator can then bring the probe across the valve and into the RV. For more advanced TV interventions 3D ICE imaging will become much more valuable.

According to the American Society of Echocardiography and the European Association of Cardiovascular Imaging, the TR severity is graded as mild, moderate, and severe.[33,34] There are qualitative, semiquantitative, and quantitative parameters in the grading severity of TR. Color flow jet area greater than 10 cm^2,

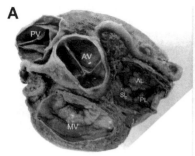 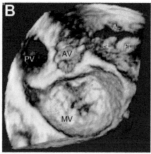

Fig. 5. Comparison of anatomic specimen (A) and 3D transesophageal echocardiography of tricuspid valve (B). MV, mitral valve; AV, aortic valve; PV, pulmonic valve.

vena contracta width 0.7 cm or more, proximal isovelocity area (PISA) radius greater than 0.9 cm, effective regurgitant orifice area (EROA) 0.4 cm^2 or more, and regurgitant volume 45 mL or greater are consistent with severe TR. The 3D PISA method is more precise than 2D PISA for determining EROA due to the noncircular orifice or eccentric TR jet.[33,35,36] Hahn and Zamorano[37] have proposed expanding the severe TR grading to massive and torrential grading as this has been shown to predict outcomes in severe patients with TR accurately.[38]

Assessment of RV dimension and function is more difficult than LV due to its conical shape in the longitudinal plane and crescent shape in the sagittal plane. RV consists of 3 parts: inlet (TA), apical (trabecular), and outlet (end at the pulmonic valve). Although cardiovascular magnetic resonance (CMR) is the goal standard method for quantification of RV size, function, and remodeling, echocardiography remains an initial method of choice. Basal diameter 4 mm or greater, midventricular diameter 35 mm or greater, or base-to-apex length 86 mm or greater indicates RV dilation.[22,39] Owing to the complex morphology, there are several surrogates of RV systolic function assessing by echocardiography. TA planar systolic excursion less than 17 mm, fractional area change less than 35%, TA systolic velocity wave (S′) measured by

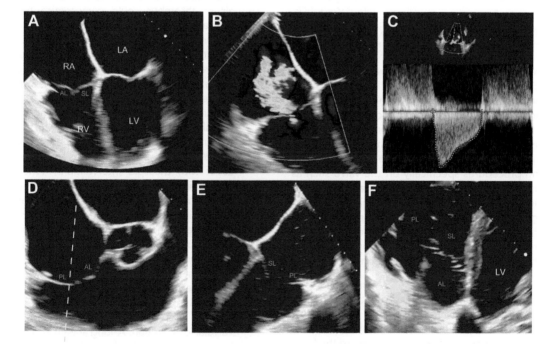

Fig. 6. Transesophageal echocardiography of tricuspid valve. (A) Midesophageal 4-chamber view at 0° demonstrating anterior and septal leaflets. (B) Color jet area. (C) Severe tricuspid regurgitation on continuous wave Doppler. (D) Midesophageal intercommissural view at 67° showing anterior and posterior leaflets. (E) Septal and posterior leaflets are seen when bringing the cursor toward the lateral, the orthogonal view (X-plane). (F) Deep gastric view providing simultaneous visualization of all 3 leaflets. LA, left atrium.

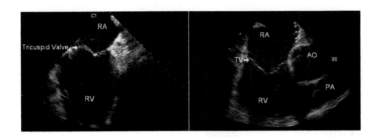

Fig. 7. Intracardiac echocardiography (ICE). TV, tricuspid valve; AO, aorta; PA, pulmonary artery.

Doppler tissue image less than 9.5 cm/s, Tei index greater than 0.43 (by pulse wave Doppler) and greater than 0.54 (by Doppler tissue imaging), and RV free wall strain greater than −20% are suggestive of RV dysfunction.[40]

Computed tomography (CT) has become a tool of choice for assessing patient eligibility and device sizing for trans-catheter tricuspid valve implant. CT imaging can provide not only target site identification, spatial relationship with RCA, and assessment of vessel planning but also optimization of fluoroscopic C-arm angulations. CT provides detailed anatomy of the IVC-RA connection. This area is an underappreciated blind spot for transcatheter procedures, but CT can identify tortuosity of the IVC, irregular IVC-RA connections, and prominent eustachian ridges. Chiari networks are better seen by echocardiography.

IMPLICATIONS FOR TRANSCATHETER TRICUSPID VALVE INTERVENTION

An important consideration when performing transcatheter TV intervention is the SVC and IVC relationship to the RA, the valve, the RV, and the right ventricular outflow tract (RVOT). The implication is that when performing procedures on the right side of the heart, usually the apparatus traverses the TV. Even when performing procedures specifically on the valve such as tricuspid edge-to-edge repair or valve implantation, the catheters, wires, and delivery sheaths follow the anatomy described previously. For the purpose of this discussion, the focus is primarily on normal anatomy without congenital malformation or surgical alteration.

- The SVC enters the RA superiorly and posteriorly; it tends to point the direction of flow toward the TV. On the contrary, the IVC enters the RA from the posterior inferior aspect and points toward the fossa ovalis. In addition, significant variability in the Chiari network directing blood across the TV from the IVC can complicate device maneuvering into the RA and across the

valve. It is for that reason that crossing into the RV or RVOT from the internal jugular approach is convenient. An example of the ease of delivering devices from the jugular approach when compared with the femoral approach is the use of RV assist devices. Delivery of the right-sided Impella (Abiomed, Danvers, Massachusetts, USA) is more difficult than implementing the ProTek Duo (LivaNova, London, England). The latter is a 29F dual-stage cannula that draws blood from the RA and pumps it directly into the pulmonary artery.

- As more large-bore procedures are performed from the IVC, operators should be mindful of patent foramen ovale (PFO) and right-side pacing leads. With multiple exchanges of large devices, embolism of air or thrombus could compromise the clinical results of procedures, therefore screening and characterization for PFO should be performed. In addition, pacemaker-related thrombus in the context of PFOs has been implicated in strokes and should be screened as well.[41]
- As annular dilation is the primary mechanism of malcoaptation for most severe TR and the RV, an anterior cardiac structure, there are chest/RV free wall interactions that can assist with tricuspid interventions. When performing procedures that require approximating opposing leaflets such as valve clipping when there is significant leaflet separation, anterior pressure at the center of the chest at the time of the procedure can help appose the leaflets and assist with capturing.
- When performing RV sample biopsy, care must be taken to avoid injuring the TV or chordal apparatus causing significant valvular dysfunction. A long sheath should be used toward the intraventricular septum and exposure of the bioptome to the valve apparatus should be minimized.
- Owing to the separation of the valve from the RVOT as described previously,

devices placed in the TA have a low risk of inducing RVOT obstruction or interfering with the pulmonic valve unlike devices implanted in the mitral position.

- When crossing the TV, it is also prudent to be aware of the location of the RA appendage, the His bundle, and the CS. It is possible to advance devices into any of those structures depending on the approach, and heart block can result from His bundle interaction.

- The TV itself is quite fragile compared with the other valves of the heart. The leaflets also deflect further so when crossing the valve care should be taken when using stiffer wires or devices, and especially while using large-bore devices such as sheaths, AngioVac (AngioDynamics, Latham, NY, USA), or valve delivery catheters. Owing to the compliance of the valve, devices such as pacemaker or ICD leads can significantly impact leaflet coaptation.

- The most common cause of TV regurgitation is annular dilation. Volume status has a profound effect on the function of the valve and appearance of pathology due to the compliance of the RV. Diuresis and medical optimization can change tricuspid annular and RV dimensions. For patients who require more ventricular depth for a transcatheter valve procedure, volume loading can improve ventricular dimensions. In patients with very large dimensions that are borderline big for devices, volume unloading can reduce RV and TV annular dimensions.

- As the annulus is complex and variable, transcatheter valves will require fixation mechanisms to anchor to the leaflets. Leaflet pathology can vary. Any combination of annular dilation, leaflet tethering, and prolapse can occur. Extreme leaflet tethering may make leaflet capture very challenging because the devices may interact with the myocardium and fail to grasp the leaflet. Furthermore, distance of the papillary muscle heads from the valvular plane can impact leaflet grasping by fixation devices. These details should be explored during patient screening.

- In procedures using percutaneous annuloplasty, anchor insertion in the TV annulus will require detailed knowledge of the relative location of the RCA to avoid coronary injury.

- The RV is highly trabeculated, and so, when placing a guide wire across the valve, the wire landing zone will depend on the depth of the RV and degree of heavy trabeculation. Coaxial trajectory through the centroid of the TA is important in the deployment of orthotopic heart valves. Careful placement of the preformed wires in the apex among the trabeculation/moderator band is a key step in orthotopic valve implantation because it assists with coaxial wire trajectory and optimizing depth for appropriate valve deployment.

- Chiari networks and prominent eustachian valves can bias or interact with procedural apparatus. Identification during screening is important.

- As with the left side, careful assessment of the RV function and pulmonary vascular resistance is necessary when performing interventions on the TV. Similar to the relationship between the mitral valve and left ventricle, correcting regurgitant TVs may reveal RV systolic dysfunction and in extreme cases, can be the cause of hemodynamic embarrassment.

- When performing transesophageal-guided procedures such as clipping, the anterior location of the TV makes it more difficult to visualize all aspects of the valve. At times, prosthetic materials (ie, mechanical aortic valve) or a lipomatous atrial septum can cause shadowing. Transgastric, 3D, and intracardiac imaging (ICE) all may help visualize the anatomy better. Use of a long sheath aimed toward the intraventricular septum may reduce the risk of TV injury during RV biopsy procedures.

SUMMARY

To safely plan and conduct transcatheter procedures on the right side of the heart a complete understanding of the TV is necessary as is an appreciation of the surrounding anatomy. As devices evolve, the nuances of device implantation from alignment to fixation will require intimate knowledge of tricuspid anatomy and the limitations of right heart physiology. Future advances in tricuspid interventions will still build upon the foundational knowledge, and simulation will play a major role in selecting interventions. The accuracy in mimicking not only the structures but also the thickness and tensile strength of the tissues will be important for planning and individualized device testing.

CLINICS CARE POINTS

- Understanding the anatomy surrounding the tricuspid valve and prior surgery modifying it allows for effective selection among the therapy options including transcatheter ones.

- The two principal causes for tricuspid valve dysfunction are annular dilation and tethering of the valve leaflets. Right ventricular remodeling due to factors such as pulmonary embolism, infarct, pulmonary hypertension, has a direct impact on tricuspid valve dysfunction.

- Imaging of the tricuspid valve is challenging due to its orientation relative to the chest and esophagus and intra-procedural transesophageal echocardiography may not show all aspects of the valve. Intra-cardiac echo may be an option in some cases.

- Evaluation of the pulmonary and right heart pressures and hemodynamics should be done as part of tricuspid valve assessment.

- The interior vena cava, enhanced by the Eustachian valve, directs blood flow towards the intra-atrial septum while the superior vena cava directs flow downwards into the right atrium. This impacts how the valve is approached and crossed using different devices.

ACKNOWLEDGMENTS

The authors would like to thank Dr Kasem Puwiwattanangkura from Plastic and Reconstructive Surgery at Faculty of Medicine, Ramathibodi Hospital, Mahidol University, Bangkok, Thailand, for the hand drawings.

DISCLOSURE

I. Abudayyeh: Edwards Lifesciences: Transcatheter valve proctor. W.L. Gore & Associates: Physician education consultant.

REFERENCES

1. Davidson LJ, Davidson CJ. Transcatheter treatment of valvular heart disease: a review. JAMA 2021; 325(24):2480–94.
2. Brauwald NS, Ross J, Morrow AG. Conservative management of tricuspid regurgitation in patients undergoing mitral valve replacement. Circulation 1967;35. I-63–I-69.
3. Demir OM, Regazzoli D, Mangieri A, et al. Transcatheter tricuspid valve replacement: principles and design. Front Cardiovasc Med 2018;5:129.
4. Singh JP, Evans JC, Levy D, et al. Prevalence and clinical determinants of mitral, tricuspid, and aortic regurgitation (the Framingham Heart Study). Am J Cardiol 1999;83(6):897–902.
5. Prihadi EA, Delgado V, Leon MB, et al. Morphologic types of tricuspid regurgitation: characteristics and prognostic implications. JACC Cardiovasc Imaging 2019;12(3):491–9.
6. Wang N, Fulcher J, Abeysuriya N, et al. Tricuspid regurgitation is associated with increased mortality independent of pulmonary pressures and right heart failure: a systematic review and meta-analysis. Eur Heart J 2019;40(5):476–84.
7. Nishimura RA, Otto CM, Bonow RO, et al. 2017 AHA/ACC focused update of the 2014 AHA/ACC guideline for the management of patients with valvular heart disease: a report of the American College of Cardiology/American Heart Association Task Force on Clinical Practice Guidelines. Circulation 2017;135(25):e1159–95.
8. Baumgartner H, Falk V, Bax JJ, et al. 2017 ESC/EACTS Guidelines for the management of valvular heart disease. Eur Heart J 2017;38(36):2739–91.
9. Westaby S, Karp RB, Blackstone EH, et al. Adult human valve dimensions and their surgical significance. Am J Cardiol 1984;53(4):552–6.
10. Holda MK, Zhingre Sanchez JD, Bateman MG, et al. Right atrioventricular valve leaflet morphology redefined: implications for transcatheter repair procedures. JACC Cardiovasc Interv 2019;12(2):169–78.
11. Ancona F, Stella S, Taramasso M, et al. Multimodality imaging of the tricuspid valve with implication for percutaneous repair approaches. Heart 2017; 103(14):1073–81.
12. Dahou A, Levin D, Reisman M, et al. Anatomy and physiology of the tricuspid valve. JACC Cardiovasc Imaging 2019;12(3):458–68.
13. Xanthos T, Dalivigkas I, Ekmektzoglou KA. Anatomic variations of the cardiac valves and papillary muscles of the right heart. Ital J Anat Embryol 2011;116(2): 111–26.
14. Rogers JH, Bolling SF. The tricuspid valve: current perspective and evolving management of tricuspid regurgitation. Circulation 2009;119(20):2718–25.
15. Muraru D, Guta AC, Ochoa-Jimenez RC, et al. Functional regurgitation of atrioventricular valves and atrial fibrillation: an elusive pathophysiological link deserving further attention. J Am Soc Echocardiogr 2020;33(1):42–53.
16. Tornos Mas P, Rodriguez-Palomares JF, Antunes MJ. Secondary tricuspid valve regurgitation: a forgotten entity. Heart 2015;101(22):1840–8.
17. Fukuda S, Saracino G, Matsumura Y, et al. Three-dimensional geometry of the tricuspid annulus in healthy subjects and in patients with functional tricuspid regurgitation: a real-time, 3-dimensional

echocardiographic study. Circulation 2006;114(1 Suppl):I492–8.

18. van Rosendael PJ, Kamperidis V, Kong WK, et al. Computed tomography for planning transcatheter tricuspid valve therapy. Eur Heart J 2017;38(9): 665–74.

19. Jokinen JJ, Turpeinen AK, Pitkanen O, et al. Pacemaker therapy after tricuspid valve operations: implications on mortality, morbidity, and quality of life. Ann Thorac Surg 2009;87(6):1806–14.

20. Bhatnagar KP, Nettleton GS, Campbell FR, et al. Chiari anomalies in the human right atrium. Clin Anat 2006;19(6):510–6.

21. Frescura C, Angelini A, Daliento L, et al. Morphological aspects of Ebstein's anomaly in adults. Thorac Cardiovasc Surg 2000;48(4):203–8.

22. Rodes-Cabau J, Taramasso M, O'Gara PT. Diagnosis and treatment of tricuspid valve disease: current and future perspectives. Lancet 2016; 388(10058):2431–42.

23. Mutlak D, Lessick J, Reisner SA, et al. Echocardiography-based spectrum of severe tricuspid regurgitation: the frequency of apparently idiopathic tricuspid regurgitation. J Am Soc Echocardiogr 2007;20(4):405–8.

24. Topilsky Y, Maltais S, Medina Inojosa J, et al. Burden of tricuspid regurgitation in patients diagnosed in the community setting. JACC Cardiovasc Imaging 2019;12(3):433–42.

25. Hoke U, Auger D, Thijssen J, et al. Significant lead-induced tricuspid regurgitation is associated with poor prognosis at long-term follow-up. Heart 2014;100(12):960–8.

26. Chang JD, Manning WJ, Ebrille E, et al. Tricuspid valve dysfunction following pacemaker or cardioverter-defibrillator implantation. J Am Coll Cardiol 2017;69(18):2331–41.

27. Kobza R, Kurz DJ, Oechslin EN, et al. Aberrant tendinous chords with tethering of the tricuspid leaflets: a congenital anomaly causing severe tricuspid regurgitation. Heart 2004;90(3):319–23.

28. Santalo-Corcoy M, Asmarats L, Li CH, et al. Catheter-based treatment of tricuspid regurgitation: state of the art. Ann Transl Med 2020;8(15):964.

29. Chang CC, Veen KM, Hahn RT, et al. Uncertainties and challenges in surgical and trans catheter tricuspid valve therapy: a state-of-the-art expert review. Our Heart J 2020;41(20):1932–40.

30. Addetia K, Yamat M, Mediratta A, et al. Comprehensive two-dimensional interrogation of the tricuspid valve using knowledge derived from three-dimensional echocardiography. J Am Soc Echocardiogr 2016;29(1):74–82.

31. Anwar AM, Geleijnse ML, Soliman OI, et al. Assessment of normal tricuspid valve anatomy in adults by real-time three-dimensional echocardiography. Int J Cardiovasc Imaging 2007;23(6):717–24.

32. Puchalski MD, Lui GK, Miller-Hance WC, et al. Guidelines for performing a comprehensive transesophageal echocardiographic: examination in children and all patients with congenital heart disease: recommendations from the American Society of Echocardiography. J Am Soc Echocardiogr 2019;32(2):173–215.

33. Zoghbi WA, Adams D, Bonow RO, et al. Recommendations for noninvasive evaluation of native valvular regurgitation: a report from the american society of echocardiography developed in collaboration with the society for cardiovascular magnetic resonance. J Am Soc Echocardiogr 2017;30(4): 303–71.

34. Lancellotti P, Tribouilloy C, Hagendorff A, et al. Recommendations for the echocardiographic assessment of native valvular regurgitation: an executive summary from the European Association of Cardiovascular Imaging. Eur Heart J Cardiovasc Imaging 2013;14(7):611–44.

35. de Agustin JA, Viliani D, Vieira C, et al. Proximal isovelocity surface area by single-beat three-dimensional color Doppler echocardiography applied for tricuspid regurgitation quantification. J Am Soc Echocardiogr 2013;26(9):1063–72.

36. Hahn RT, Thomas JD, Khalique OK, et al. Imaging assessment of tricuspid regurgitation severity. JACC Cardiovasc Imaging 2019;12(3): 469–90.

37. Hahn RT, Zamorano JL. The need for a new tricuspid regurgitation grading scheme. Eur Heart J Cardiovasc Imaging 2017;18(12):1342–3.

38. Fortuni F, Dietz MF, Butcher SC, et al. Prognostic implications of increased right ventricular wall tension in secondary tricuspid regurgitation. Am J Cardiol 2020;136:131–9.

39. Correa-Villasenor A, Ferencz C, Neill CA, et al. Ebstein's malformation of the tricuspid valve: genetic and environmental factors. The Baltimore-Washington Infant Study Group. Teratology 1994; 50(2):137–47.

40. Lang RM, Badano LP, Mor-Avi V, et al. Recommendations for cardiac chamber quantification by echocardiography in adults: an update from the American Society of Echocardiography and the European Association of Cardiovascular Imaging. J Am Soc Echocardiogr 2015;28(1):1–39.e14.

41. DeSimone CV, Friedman PA, Noheria A, et al. Stroke or transient ischemic attack in patients with trans venous pacemaker or defibrillator and echocardiographically detected patient foramen ovale. Circulation 2013;128(13):1433–41.

Echocardiographic Imaging of the Tricuspid Valve

Preprocedural Planning and Intraprocedural Guidance

Pradhum Ram, MD[a], Nikoloz Shekiladze, MD[a], Joe Xie, MD[a,b], Patrick T. Gleason, MD[a,b,*]

KEYWORDS

• Transcatheter tricuspid valve interventions • Interventional echo • Tricuspid regurgitation

KEY POINTS

- Imaging of the tricuspid valve is challenging and often requires a multimodality imaging approach.
- Transesophageal imaging can be difficult to obtain due to shadowing from mitral or aortic prosthesis as well as intracardiac device wires.
- Advances in multiplanar transesophageal echocardiography have improved our ability to perform transcatheter tricuspid valve procedures.

 Video content accompanies this article at http://www.interventional.theclinics.com

INTRODUCTION

Interest in transcatheter therapies for tricuspid valve (TV) disease has accelerated in recent years given increased recognition and poor prognosis associated with severe tricuspid regurgitation (TR).[1–4] Concurrent with the evolution of transcatheter strategies to treat TR, the need for multimodality imaging support has also grown tremendously. In particular, the ability to provide comprehensive echocardiographic (echo) imaging of the TV both preprocedure and intraprocedure has become critical to procedural success.[5–8] In this article, the authors aim to cover key aspects of both preprocedural and intraprocedural echo imaging.

PREPROCEDURE PLANNING

Preprocedure echo provides insight into the anatomy and cause of TR in order to determine possible strategies for repair versus replacement.[7] Anatomically, the TV comprises several components—the leaflets, subvalvular apparatus, and the annulus—similar to the structural composition of the mitral valve. There are 3 TV leaflets (anterior, posterior, and septal) with significant variations in leaflet size, shape, and chordal attachments. In general, the anterior leaflet has the largest area with the greatest mobility; the posterior leaflet (occasionally multiscalloped) has the smallest circumferential distance, and the septal leaflet has the shortest radial distance. The septal leaflet is also the least mobile and frequently has chordae that attach directly to the interventricular septum. As such, there are usually 2 distinct papillary muscles (anterior and posterior) with a variable septal papillary muscle. The anatomic position of the leaflets can also differ among patients; however, the anterior-septal commissure is

[a] Division of Cardiology, Emory University Hospital, 550 Peachtree Street NE, 4th Floor, Davis-Fischer Building, Atlanta, GA 30308, USA; [b] Division of Cardiology, Emory Structural Heart and Valve Center, 550 Peachtree Street NE, 4th Floor, Davis-Fischer Building, Atlanta, GA 30308, USA
* Corresponding author. Division of Cardiology, Emory Structural Heart and Valve Center, 550 Peachtree Street, 4th floor Davis-Fischer Building, Atlanta, GA 30308, USA.
E-mail addresses: pgleaso@emory.edu; patrick.t.gleason@emory.edu

Intervent Cardiol Clin 11 (2022) 11–25
https://doi.org/10.1016/j.iccl.2021.09.001
2211-7458/22/© 2021 Elsevier Inc. All rights reserved.

typically located near the noncoronary cusp of the aortic valve, and the posterior-septal commissure is adjacent to the entrance of the coronary sinus within the right atrium (RA). The anterior-posterior commissure can be difficult to visualize and is not always anatomically distinct. Finally, the TV annulus is a complex and highly dynamic structure that changes significantly with loading conditions. The annulus is usually described as saddle shaped with a more superiorly displaced anteroseptal aspect and a more inferiorly positioned posteroseptal side of the annulus. In cases of annular dilation, the septal leaflet is typically protected by the muscular interventricular septum, and thus, dilation occurs mostly along the anterior and posterior leaflets leading to a more circular and planar TV annulus.[5–7]

Broadly, TR can be classified as either primary or secondary TR. Primary, or degenerative, TR is rare and caused by an acquired or congenital pathologic condition of the leaflets and/or chords. Secondary or "functional" TR comprises most cases of TR and can be due to left-sided heart disease, pulmonary hypertension, right ventricular (RV) dysfunction and dilation, or idiopathic causes without a primary defect of the TV itself.

When considering transcatheter therapies, secondary TR can generally be described as either (1) dilatation of the annulus owing to enlargement of the RV and RA, or (2) tethering and restriction of the TV leaflets. Understanding the underlying pathophysiology determines the target for transcatheter devices (ie, annulus vs leaflet strategies).[9,10] In addition, RV size and function, pulmonary pressures, the presence of any pacemaker or implantable cardioverter-defibrillator (ICD) leads, and subvalvular structures are additional important considerations during procedural planning. Transthoracic echocardiography (TTE) and transesophageal echocardiography (TEE) are complementary in evaluating the TV and provide critical information in understanding the complex mechanism of TR. Both the American Society of Echocardiography and the European Society of Cardiology guidelines provide a comprehensive list of recommended views needed for TV visualization.[11–15] The authors have summarized a few important views in later discussion.

TRANSTHORACIC ECHOCARDIOGRAPHY VIEWS

Identification of the individual leaflets is challenging given the anatomic variability of the TV and highly dependent on the angulation of the transducer. In general, from the parasternal inflow view, the near-field leaflet is usually the anterior leaflet (Fig. 1). The far-field leaflet can be either the septal leaflet if the coronary sinus ostium or intraventricular septum (IVS) is seen, or the posterior leaflet if these landmarks are not concurrently visualized[10] (see Fig. 1).

In the parasternal short axis at the level of the aortic valve, a single large anterior leaflet is often seen. If 2 leaflets are visualized, there are usually the anterior (adjacent to the aortic valve) and posterior leaflets. If the left ventricular outflow tract (LVOT) is seen instead of the aortic valve, the TV leaflets are likely the septal (adjacent to the LVOT) and posterior leaflets (Fig. 2).[10]

From the apical views, the septal leaflet is seen adjacent to the IVS, and the opposing leaflet can be either the anterior or the posterior leaflet. With an anterior angulation toward the LVOT, the septal and anterior leaflets are typically identified. With a more posterior angulation toward the coronary sinus, the septal and posterior leaflets can be seen (Fig. 3).[10]

Notably, all 3 TV leaflets are rarely seen at the same time by a 2-dimensional (2D) TTE imaging plane but can be better visualized with 3-dimensional (3D) imaging. Given the anterior position of the TV and right heart, 3D TTE images are sometimes better in quality than 3D TEE. Multiple volumes from the different views should still be captured and include adjacent landmarks to accurately identify each leaflet.

TRANSESOPHAGEAL ECHOCARDIOGRAPHY VIEWS

Similar to TTE evaluation of the TV, the assessment by TEE also requires multiple depths and angulations and includes the midesophageal, deep esophageal, and transgastric views. 3D volumes should be obtained at each position.

Starting in the midesophageal position at 0°, the septal leaflet is seen adjacent to the IVS in the standard 4-chamber view (Table 1). The opposing leaflet is typically the anterior leaflet if the probe is anteflexed or the posterior leaflet if retroflexed. The midesophageal inflow-outflow view can be obtained by increasing the transducer angle to 60° to 90°. With the short axis of the aortic valve in view, the TV leaflets in view are the anterior (adjacent to the aortic valve) and posterior leaflets. An "X-plane" or simultaneous biplane through the anterior or posterior leaflet will allow visualization of the

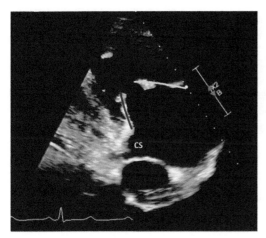

Fig. 1. Parasternal RV-inflow view ("hip-shot") demonstrating TV leaflets in long axis (*red*) septal leaflet and (*yellow*) anterior leaflet. CS, coronary sinus.

septal leaflet along with the anterior or posterior leaflet, respectively (see Table 1). This inflow-outflow view can also provide the most parallel Doppler angle for optimal continuous-wave and pulse-wave Doppler measurements.

Advancing the probe from either the 4-chamber view at 0° or the inflow-outflow view will produce the corresponding deep esophageal images. The left-sided heart structures will typically disappear from the near field and can produce less obstructed views of the TV. The same biplane and Doppler evaluation of the TV should be performed in the deep esophageal views. Whether in the midesophagus or deep esophagus, the inflow-outflow view with simultaneous biplane usually allows the most detailed

assessment of leaflet anatomy, coaptation, and chordal structures from the esophagus.

Further advancement of the probe into the stomach will produce the transgastric views of the TV. Slowly increasing the transducer angle to 30° to 60° with rightward rotation of the probe will produce the short-axis view of the TV. In this image, the septal leaflet is adjacent to the IVS; the posterior leaflet is in the near field, and the anterior leaflet is in the far field. A horizontal long-axis view of the RA and RV with the TV orthogonal to the imaging plane can be visualized with the transducer angle at 0°; however, it can more reliably be obtained by increasing the transducer angle further to 90° to 120° with a rightward or "clocked" rotation. The septal leaflet will disappear from the image, and the posterior leaflet will remain in the near field with the anterior leaflet in the far field. Biplane through these leaflet tips will again reproduce the short axis of the TV. Visualization of an en face short axis of the TV provides complementary information to the images obtained in the midesophagus and deep esophagus and can precisely determine the location of any mal-coaptation between leaflets, identify leaflet morphology as well as papillary muscles and chordal attachments (see Table 1).

DETERMINATION OF TRANSCATHETER OPTIONS

Based on patient characteristics and imaging findings, a determination is made if the patient is eligible for surgery, transcatheter approach, or ineligible for any TV procedure. If transcatheter therapies are considered, the preprocedure echo and computed tomographic (CT) imagings are critical to understanding the options for treatment. A TV with dense chordal attachments to the leaflet tips, large coaptation or flail gap (>10 mm), severely restricted leaflets, or pacemaker/ICD leads impinging on the TV leaflets are typically unfavorable characteristics for TV transcatheter edge-to-edge repair (TEER). Transcatheter tricuspid valve replacement (TTVR) is typically more feasible in these patients as well as in patients with large TV annulus size; however, CT preplanning and manufacturing specifications are essential to ensuring an appropriate device selection.

INTRAPROCEDURAL GUIDANCE FOR TRANSCATHETER THERAPIES

With the growth of transcatheter TV devices, the knowledge and tools used for procedural

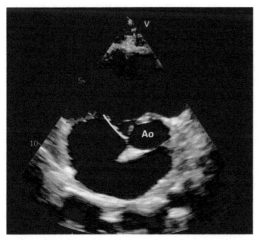

Fig. 2. Parasternal short-axis view of TV visualizing anterior (*yellow*) and posterior (*blue*) leaflets. Ao, aorta.

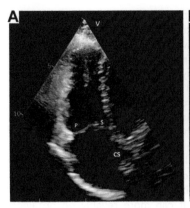 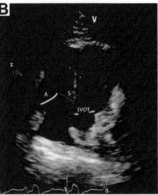

Fig. 3. Four-apical view of TV: (A) Inferiorly angled view demonstrating posterior (blue) and septal (red) leaflets. (B) Anteriorly angled view demonstrating anterior (yellow) and septal (red) leaflets. A, anterior leaflet; P, posterior leaflet; S, septal leaflet.

guidance have advanced tremendously. Although intraprocedure guidance of transcatheter TV therapies currently relies mostly on TEE, there are select cases whereby TEE image quality is poor and TTE and/or intracardiac echo (ICE) may offer helpful adjunctive images.[10,16] Current ICE technology is limited, and more advanced 3D ICE is currently in development. In this section, the authors focus on TEE image guidance.

As with any transcatheter procedure, it is important to start with the 4-chamber view. The 4-chamber view is important because it allows for assessment of global left ventricular (LV) and RV size and function, left atrium (LA) and RA size, and whether there is a preexisting pericardial effusion. For transcatheter TV interventions, an RV-focused view is needed to evaluate the RV function, which can be impacted perioperatively.

Similar to the preprocedure echo, the authors recommend a thorough evaluation of the TV leaflets and degree of regurgitation. This is best accomplished by looking at the TV with and without color Doppler in multiple views, including the 4-chamber view, RV inflow-outflow view, deep esophageal view, and the transgastric view. Biplane imaging is critical to understand the morphology of the valve leaflets, the size and location of the regurgitant jet or jets, and subvalvular structures. Last, depending on what procedure is performed, 3D images of the TV may be necessary for valve alignment and deployment, so establishing where the optimal windows are is important to procedural success.[16–19]

IMAGING FOR LEAFLET COAPTATION DEVICES

TEER technology has been used on the mitral valve successfully for several years. Although there are no commercially available devices for TEER for the TV, there are several in clinical trials that share many of the same features, and from an intraprocedural imaging perspective are very similar.

Preprocedure, the interventional imager should have an idea of the leaflets and location, which will be targeted for approximation during the procedure based on the preprocedural imaging as described above.

At the beginning of the procedure, the wires and guide catheter will be advanced into the RA under echo guidance from either a bicaval view or a 3D view. After the guide is placed in the RA, the device delivery catheter will be advanced through the guide. As the device delivery catheter is advanced out of the guide, the interventional cardiologist will start to steer the system down toward the TV. It is important to monitor this step either in 3D using multiplanar reconstruction (MPR) or more commonly from the RV inflow-outflow view with biplane imaging (Fig. 4). The goal of the initial catheter placement would be to ensure that the delivery catheter is away from the interatrial septum and has a relatively straight and coaxial alignment to the TV in the biplane image. Once that correct trajectory is confirmed, attention can be turned to lining up the device to the correct location on the valve where the leaflet will be grasped (Fig. 5). To achieve this, the imager will use the RV inflow-outflow view with biplane as well as transgastric views. In the midesophageal inflow-outflow view, moving the device catheter closer to the aortic valve brings the device into an anterior/septal location. Moving more toward the RV free wall in this view takes the device toward the posterior septal location. Rotation of the device so that the arms or "wings" of the device are seen in the orthogonal view from the inflow-outflow view is then

Table 1
Transesophageal echocardiography tricuspid valve imaging: important views from preprocedure to device implant

A. Four-chamber evaluation for pericardial effusion	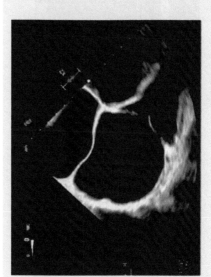
B. RV-focused view: assess RV size and function before the procedure	

(continued on next page)

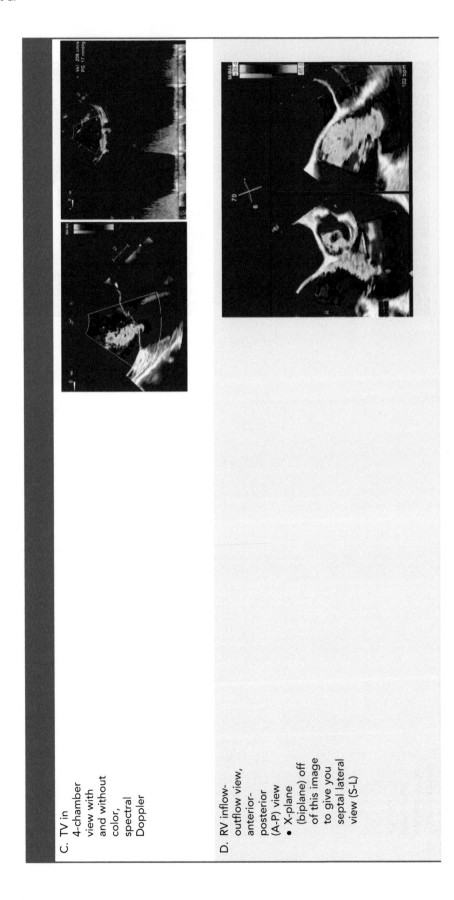

C. TV in 4-chamber view with and without color, spectral Doppler

D. RV inflow-outflow view, anterior-posterior (A-P) view
- X-plane (biplane) off of this image to give you septal lateral view (S-L)

E. Transgastric
views
- Long and
  short axis
  of the
  tricuspid
  valve
- Aortic Valve
  and LVOT
  spectral Doppler

F. 3D TEE:
- Aorta
  rotated to
  the left part
  of the
  screen in
  the anatomic
  "surgeon's
  view"

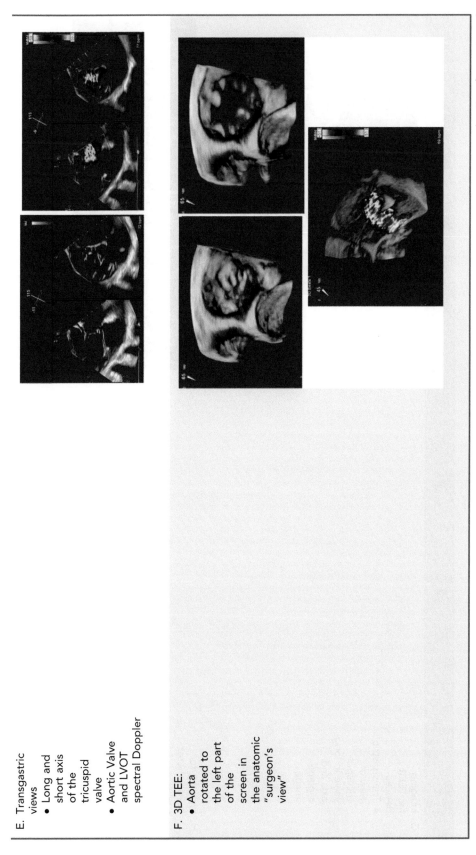

(continued on next page)

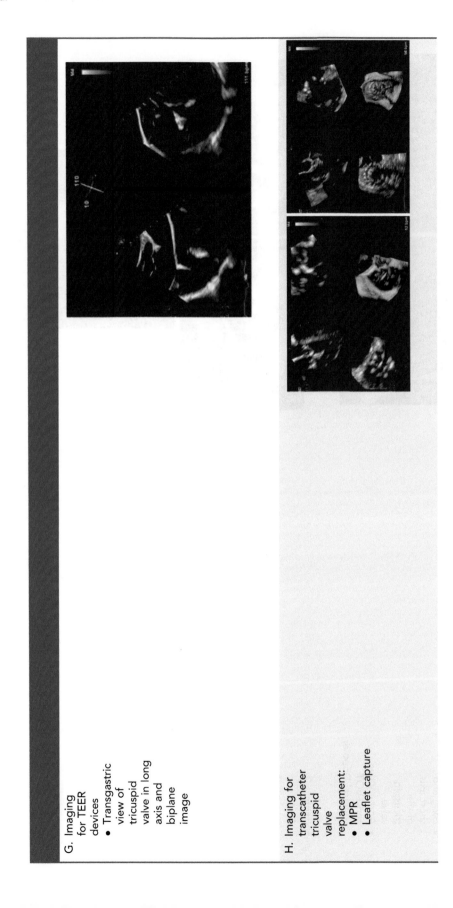

G. Imaging
   for TEER
   devices
   • Transgastric
     view of
     tricuspid
     valve in long
     axis and
     biplane
     image

H. Imaging for
   transcatheter
   tricuspid
   valve
   replacement:
   • MPR
   • Leaflet capture

I. Imaging for annuloplasty devices and other novel procedures:
- MPR: tricuspid annulus

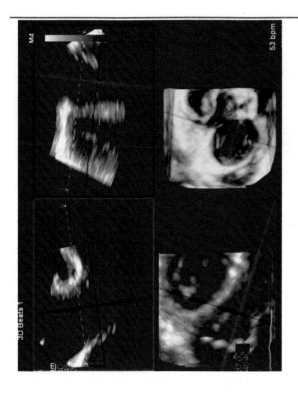

J. Imaging for valve in valve or valve in ring:
- Four-chamber view of tricuspid bioprosthetic valve

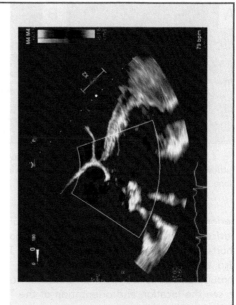

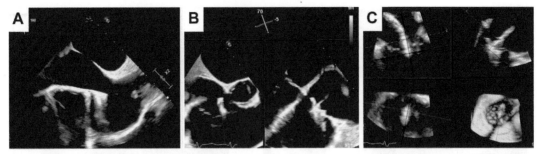

Fig. 4. (*A*) TEE bicaval view demonstrating a device delivery catheter steering down to TV. (*B*, *C*) TEE RV inflow-outflow view with biplane image and MPR showing safe and accurate delivery of the TEER system in the annular plane.

performed. The position and orientation of the device are then confirmed in the transgastric short-axis views. A long-axis view of the TV is also obtained, and biplane is used to scan through the valve from tip to annulus in order to see the location and orientation of the TEER device (seeFig. 5).

After confirming the location and orientation of the device is appropriate, the device can be advanced into the RV under echo guidance from the midesophageal RV inflow-outflow view with biplane. Once under the TV leaflets, the focus is turned to leaflet capture. A zoomed-in view of the device arms and interaction with the leaflets is helpful at this stage of the procedure. To properly capture the leaflets, the leaflet should lie down on top of the TEER device arm, reaching the central body of the device (Fig. 6). The imager should see restricted leaflet motion, which will further support adequate capture. Given that the current generation TEER devices have independent grasping function, each leaflet is grasped separately, that is, the anterior leaflet is first grasped followed by the septal leaflet. Once the leaflets have been grasped, device orientation and location are confirmed in the transgastric view before closing the device arms. During this check, the length of the leaflet capture is also noted and confirmed that the leaflet is inserted to the central body of the device. After confirmation of location and orientation of the grasp, the device is moved into the "closed" position with the grasped leaflets (Fig. 7). Visualization of the leaflets in the midesophageal inflow-outflow view with biplane as well as transgastric view confirms that the leaflets have not moved. Color Doppler is then used to see if there has been an impact on the degree of TR. If the color Doppler shows improvement in the degree of TR, then the device is usually deployed, and a decision is made regarding the need for a second clip. A second clip is introduced, oriented, and delivered under the same echo-guided steps as above. If the TR has not improved or is worse, then the device arms should be moved back into the "ready or open" position. Typically, a suboptimal result on color Doppler usually requires the optimization of leaflet grasp or which can be determined based on location

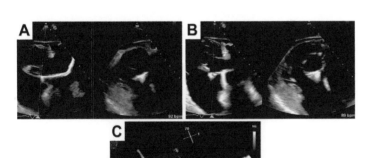

Fig. 5. TEE transgastric view of TV in long axis with biplane imaging through the leaflet tips confirming the position of the TEER device in anteroseptal orientation in systole (*A*) and diastole (*B*). (*C*) RV inflow-outflow view with biplane image showing anterior and septal leaflets.

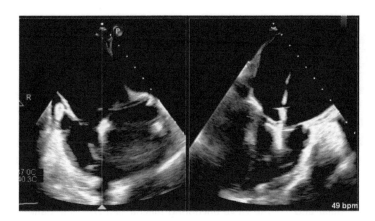

Fig. 6. TEE RV inflow-outflow view with biplane demonstrating leaflet proper capture by TEER.

and orientation. Small adjustments in leaflet grasp and location are made until there is improvement in the color or a new anatomic location is attempted. Before final release of the device, the mean TV gradient needs to be measured to make sure that there is no significant TV stenosis. The mean TV gradient is typically 0 to 1 mm Hg at baseline. After TEER, the mean TV would be expected to be less than 5 mm Hg, but it is usually 1 to 2 mm Hg. Once a satisfactory result is obtained, the device is released, and the imager makes a final assessment of the TV. In addition to a mean TV gradient, color Doppler should be assessed, as this can change once the device is released. Leaflet capture and device stability should also be assessed, in addition to evaluation of RV function and presence of a pericardial effusion (see **Fig. 7**).

IMAGING FOR TRICUSPID VALVE REPLACEMENT DEVICES

Although there are no commercially available transcatheter TTVR devices available at the time of this publication, there are several devices at various stages of clinical investigation. Each device has its own unique design, but they all share common features in that there is a leaflet and/or annular anchoring mechanism and an inner bioprosthetic valve. Patient eligibility for TTVR is based on several factors, including patient characteristics, annulus dimensions as determined by CT, RV function as well as manufacturer-specific device sizes. All these elements, including annular assessment by CT, are described elsewhere.

After the patient is intubated, baseline images are obtained as previously described. It is important to confirm that there has been no

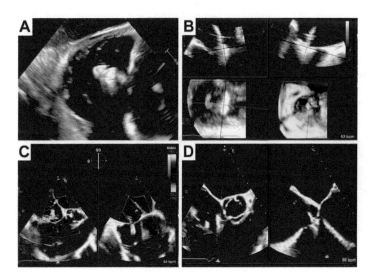

Fig. 7. (A) Transgastric TEE view of short axis TV and (B) MPR showing septal and anterior leaflet capture and approximation. (C) TEE RV inflow-outflow view with biplane demonstrating residual TR after TEER by color Doppler. (D) TEE RV inflow-outflow view with biplane showing "tissue bridge."

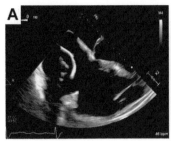
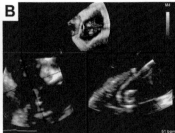
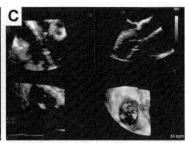

Fig. 8. (A) TEE demonstrating wire in the RA and (B) MPR showing the wire in the ventricle. (C) Confirmation of central wire location by MPR.

significant change in leaflet motion, annular and chamber size, and RV and LV function, as this may alter the plan. If a significant change is noted, such as decreased RV function or enlargement of the RV cavity, it may be prudent to abort the procedure and optimize the patient further.

As with TEER, the first step in echo guidance is the placement of a guide catheter into the RA, which can usually be performed using 3D with a large sector width encompassing the entire RA. If 3D resolution does not allow for this, the bicaval view can be used. Once the guide catheter is placed centrally in the RA and directed toward the TV, a wire is typically introduced into the right ventricle. It is critically important that the wire is placed into the apex of the right ventricle and is centrally placed in the TV, free of chordae or entanglement in subvalvular apparatus. To ensure the wire is properly placed, it is recommended to use 3D MPR as well as transgastric long-axis views to confirm apical wire placement from multiple vantage points (Fig. 8). After the wire placement is confirmed, the valve is typically introduced into the RA and slowly advanced into the RA using 3D MPR. For the remainder of the procedure, 3D MPR will be used almost exclusively because it offers many advantages, including coaxial visualization of the tricuspid annulus, real-time location and orientation of the valve, and continuous 360° evaluation of the interaction of

the valve anchoring mechanism with the leaflets and/or annulus. As the anchoring mechanism is exposed in the RV, the en face MPR is rotated to visualize the interaction of the anchoring mechanism and leaflets as well as the annulus (Fig. 9). This requires great attention to detail to ensure all the possible leaflets are captured (Video 1). Failure to capture the leaflets will result in paravalvular leak (PVL) after release of the valve or possible device embolization. The device will be further expanded and deployed, stopping intermittently to confirm that there is proper insertion of the leaflets into the anchoring mechanism with rotation of the en face MPR. Once the anchoring mechanism is fully exposed and the device is brought up to the annulus, the transcatheter valve is then deployed with the inner valve being fully expanded rapidly. At this point, the valve is deployed, and an assessment of the final valve position and function is performed. Using a combination of midesophageal 2D with biplane, 3D MPR, and transgastric imaging with and without color Doppler, the valve is evaluated for position and orientation, leaflet function, degree of valvular regurgitation and stenosis, and PVL (Fig. 10; Videos 2 and 3). If the valve was deployed with proper sizing and alignment, it is extremely unlikely the valve would embolize or migrate.[19,20] Paravalvular regurgitation should be graded in keeping with American Society of Echocardiography guidelines.[12,13] Trace

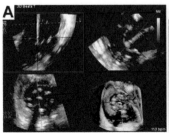
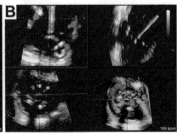

Fig. 9. (A) and (B) 3D MPR of tricuspid transcatheter valve in short axis showing location and orientation of the valve for 360° evaluation of the interaction of the valve anchoring mechanism with the leaflets and/or annulus.

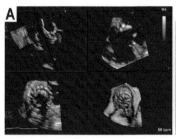
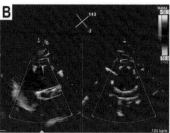

Fig. 10. (A) 3D MPR short axis of transcatheter TV postdeployment. (B) TEE long-axis view of tricuspid annulus with color Doppler posttranscatheter valve deployment demonstrating absence of residual TR.

or mild PVL is typically monitored without further intervention, whereas moderate or greater PVL may require further intervention, such as PVL leak closure or deployment of a second valve within the first valve.

IMAGING FOR TRANSCATHETER ANNULOPLASTY DEVICES

When compared with surgical TV annuloplasty, which is well established and commonly performed, transcatheter solutions for tricuspid annuloplasty are still being developed and refined. At the time of this publication, there are no devices in active enrollment for transcatheter annuloplasty devices, although several devices have been trialed and are undergoing further design changes before reintroduction. The device characteristics and implantation techniques are described elsewhere. From an imaging standpoint, transcatheter tricuspid annuloplasty device implants can be a challenging and arduous implant, as there can be up to 17 screws that need to be implanted on the atrial side of the tricuspid annulus. Each of these screws is placed under echo guidance using 3D MPR with rotation of the en face image as the device is implanted around the annulus. Once all the screws are implanted, the device is cinched down under echo guidance to reduce the anterior-posterior dimension as well as the septal-lateral dimension. While the screws are being placed, it is important to monitor for perforation of the RA wall or injury to the right coronary artery with accumulation of a pericardial effusion. In addition, once the device is implanted and cinched, the imager needs to check for dehiscence as well as note the change in TR and leaflet motion.[21]

IMAGING FOR BALLOON-EXPANDABLE TRANSCATHETER HEART VALVE IN A SURGICAL RING OR SURGICAL BIOPROSTHESIS

If there is failure or degeneration of either surgical tricuspid annuloplasty or bioprosthetic valve replacement, transcatheter valve replacement using a balloon-expandable valve within the annuloplasty or surgical valve may be an option. Preprocedure CT is critical to determine if there is a transcatheter valve replacement option and is described elsewhere. After correct sizing and approach are determined on CT, intraprocedural TEE can be used for procedural guidance, but the procedure is primarily guided by fluoroscopy because of the reliable fluoroscopic landmarks. Once the transcatheter valve is advanced, either biplane imaging or 3D MPR can be used to show if the valve is coaxial to the annulus. The valve is then deployed with rapid pacing. After deployment in an annuloplasty ring, there is a high likelihood of PVL near the septal leaflet owing to the incomplete ("U" shaped) annuloplasty rings that are commonly used in surgery. Moderate or greater PVL likely should be plugged before finishing the procedure. In tricuspid valve-in-valve procedures, if the valve was sized appropriately, PVL is typically trace or mild and does not warrant further intervention. Full assessment of the transcatheter valve should be performed using 2D and 3D with and without color Doppler as well as spectral Doppler to evaluate valve gradients.

SUMMARY

Transcatheter TV interventions have increased dramatically in recent years. TV imaging is challenging in many respects. Given the TV's anatomic complexity, multimodality imaging, which is centered on echo, plays a significant part in planning and execution of these interventions. With the help of echo-guided imaging, pathophysiologic mechanisms for TV disease are better understood, and thus, appropriate valve intervention can be strategized. Novel devices for the TV continue to be developed, and thus, intraprocedural echo imaging will continue to evolve in the days ahead.

CLINICS CARE POINTS

- Imaging of the tricuspid valve is challenging and often requires a multimodality imaging approach.
- A comprehensive transthoracic echocardiography and transesophageal echocardiography are necessary to understand potential therapies available to patients.
- In patients with dense chordal attachments to the leaflet tips, large coaptation gaps, severely restricted leaflets, and/or leaflet impingement from a pacemaker or implantable cardioverter-defibrillator, transcatheter edge-to-edge repair is challenging. These patients are likely better served with tricuspid valve replacement solutions.
- Echocardiographic 3-dimensional multiplanar reconstruction is frequently used for intraprocedural transcatheter tricuspid valve interventions because of improved visualization of the valve and the interaction with the tricuspid valve complex.

ACKNOWLEDGMENTS

Drs. Xie and Gleason's employer (Emory) has research contracts for clinical investigation of transcatheter aortic, mitral, and tricuspid devices from Edwards Lifesciences, Abbott Vascular, Medtronic, and Boston Scientific.

DISCLOSURE

The authors have no financial disclosures.

SUPPLEMENTARY DATA

Supplementary data related to this article can be found online at 10.1016/j.iccl.2021.09.001.

REFERENCES

1. Dietz MF, Prihadi EA, van der Bijl P, et al. Prognostic implications of right ventricular remodeling and function in patients with significant secondary tricuspid regurgitation. Circulation 2019;140: 836–45.
2. Fender EA, Zack CJ, Nishimura RA. Isolated tricuspid regurgitation: outcomes and therapeutic interventions. Heart 2018;104:798–806.
3. Benfari G, Antoine C, Miller WL, et al. Excess mortality associated with functional tricuspid regurgitation complicating heart failure with reduced ejection fraction. Circulation 2019;140: 196–206.
4. Wang N, Fulcher J, Abeysuriya N, et al. Tricuspid regurgitation is associated with increased mortality independent of pulmonary pressures and right heart failure: a systematic review and meta-analysis. Eur Heart J 2019;40:476–84.
5. Khalique OK, Cavalcante JL, Shah D, et al. Multimodality imaging of the tricuspid valve and right heart anatomy. JACC Cardiovasc Imaging 2019; 12:516–31.
6. Hahn RT, Thomas JD, Khalique OK, Cavalcante JL, Praz F, Zoghbi WA, et al. Imaging assessment of tricuspid regurgitation severity. JACC Cardiovasc Imaging 2019;12:469–90.
7. Prihadi EA, Delgado V, Hahn RT, Leipsic J, Min JK, Bax JJ, et al. Imaging needs in novel transcatheter tricuspid valve interventions. JACC Cardiovasc Imaging 2018;11:736–54.
8. Bartko PE, Arfsten H, Frey MK, Heitzinger G, Pavo N, Cho A, et al. Natural history of functional tricuspid regurgitation: implications of quantitative Doppler assessment. JACC Cardiovasc Imaging 2019;12:389–97.
9. Winkel MG, Brugger N, Khalique OK, et al. Imaging and patient selection for transcatheter tricuspid valve interventions. Front Cardiovasc Med 2020;7:60.
10. Hahn RT. State-of-the-art review of echocardiographic imaging in the evaluation and treatment of functional tricuspid regurgitation. Circulation 2016;9:e005332.
11. Nishimura RA, Otto CM, Bonow RO, et al. American College of Cardiology/American Heart Association Task Force on practice, AHA/ACC guideline for the management of patients with valvular heart disease: a report of the American College of Cardiology/American Heart Association Task Force on Practice Guidelines. J Am Cull Cardiol 2014;63: e57–185.
12. Rudski LG, Lai WW, Afilalo J, et al. Guidelines for the echocardiographic assessment of the right heart in adults: a report from the American Society of Echocardiography endorsed by the European Association of Echocardiography, a registered branch of the European Society of Cardiology, and the Canadian Society of Echocardiography. J Am Soc Echocardiogr 2010;23: 685–713.
13. Lang RM, Badano LP, Mor-Avi V, et al. Recommendations for cardiac chamber quantification by echocardiography in adults: an update from the American Society of Echocardiography and the European Association of Cardiovascular imaging. J Am Soc Echocardiogr 2015;28:1–39.e14.
14. Mediratta A, Addetia K, Yamat M, et al. 3D echocardiographic location of implantable device

leads and mechanism of associated tricuspid regurgitation. JACC Cardiovasc Imaging 2014;7: 337–47.

15. Addetia K, Harb SC, Hahn RT, et al. Cardiac implantable electronic device lead-induced tricuspid regurgitation. JACC Cardiovasc Imaging 2019;12:622–36.

16. Hahn RT, Abraham T, Adams MS, et al. Guidelines for performing a comprehensive transesophageal echocardiographic examination: recommendations from the American Society of Echocardiography and the Society of Cardiovascular Anesthesiologists. J Am Soc Echocardiogr 2013; 26:921–64.

17. Hahn RT. Assessment and procedural guidance with echocardiography for transcatheter tricuspid

regurgitation devices. Prog Cardiovasc Dis 2019; 62(6):452–8.

18. Muraru D, Hahn RT, Soliman OI, et al. 3-Dimensional echocardiography in imaging the tricuspid valve. JACC Cardiovasc Imaging 2019;12(3): 500–15.

19. Hahn RT, Thomas JD, Khalique OK, et al. Imaging assessment of tricuspid regurgitation severity. JACC Cardiovasc Imaging 2019;12(3):469–90.

20. Rodés-Cabau J, Hahn RT, Latib A, et al. Transcatheter therapies for treating tricuspid regurgitation. J Am Coll Cardiol 2016;67(15):1829–45.

21. Hahn RT, Nabauer M, Zuber M, et al. Intraprocedural imaging of transcatheter tricuspid valve interventions. JACC Cardiovasc Imaging 2019;12(3): 532–53.

Cardiac Computed Tomography and Magnetic Resonance Imaging of the Tricuspid Valve: Preprocedural Planning and Postprocedural Follow-up

Bernardo B.C. Lopes, MD[a], Go Hashimoto, MD[a],
Vinayak N. Bapat, MBBS[b,c], Paul Sorajja, MD[b,c],
Markus D. Scherer, MD[d], João L. Cavalcante, MD[a,b,c],*

KEYWORDS

- Tricuspid valve • Tricuspid regurgitation • Transcatheter valve intervention
- Computed tomography • Magnetic resonance

KEY POINTS

- Cardiac CT and MRI have not been traditionally used for the evaluation of TR patients, however their complementary role has been increasingly recognized.
- Dedicated imaging acquisition protocols to maximize imaging quality in this challenging group of patients, often with atrial fibrillation, intracardiac devices and/or inability to breath-hold.
- Multimodality imaging has a central role in the development, implementation, and evolution of transcatheter TR interventions, improving understanding of patient selection, procedural planning and outcomes.

 Video content accompanies this article at http://www.interventional.theclinics.com.

INTRODUCTION

Surgical treatment of isolated tricuspid regurgitation (TR) carries the highest risk of all valve surgeries.[1] Less invasive transcatheter tricuspid interventions (TTVIs) are emerging as an alternative for patients with TR.[2] Multimodality imaging has a central role in the development, implementation, and evolution of these new TR interventions.[3]

The tricuspid valve (TV) is challenging to assess. The anterior and rightward location which is in the far, lateral field from the esophagus for transesophageal echocardiography (TEE) (Fig. 1), the thin leaflets with variable anatomy, and the 3-dimensional (3D) shape of the

---

[a] Cardiovascular Imaging Research Center and Core Lab, Minneapolis Heart Institute Foundation, 920 East 28th Street, Suite 100, Minneapolis, MN 55047, USA; [b] Valve Science Center, Minneapolis Heart Institute Foundation, 920 East 28th Street, Minneapolis, MN 55047, USA; [c] Minneapolis Heart Institute, Abbott Northwestern Hospital, 920 East 28th Street, Suite 100, Minneapolis, MN 55047, USA; [d] Sanger Heart & Vascular Institute Adult Cardiology Kenilworth, 1237 Harding Place Suite 3100, Charlotte, NC 28203, USA
* Corresponding author. Minneapolis Heart Institute Foundation, 920 East 28th Street, Suite 100, Minneapolis, MN 55407
E-mail address: Joao.Cavalcante@allina.com
Twitter: @JoaoLCavalcante (J.L.C.)

Intervent Cardiol Clin 11 (2022) 27–40
https://doi.org/10.1016/j.iccl.2021.09.004

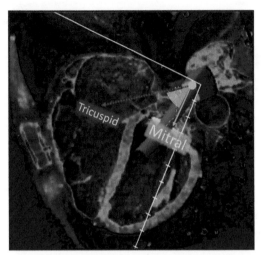

Fig. 1. TEE simulation using CCT images showing the anatomic position of the tricuspid valve in relation to the TEE probe. Compared with the mitral valve, the tricuspid valve is in the far, lateral field of view on TEE, which makes the evaluation more challenging.

annulus and the underlying right ventricle (RV) hamper conventional 2-dimensional (2D) echocardiographic evaluation.[4] The complementary role of cardiac computed tomography (CCT) and magnetic resonance (CMR) for the evaluation of patients with symptomatic TR has been increasingly recognized.[3,4] CCT has been already an integral part of TTVI planning, essential for device sizing and predicting procedural complications.

Understanding the strengths and clinical applications of each imaging modality is a requisite for the structural heart team. This review provides an updated overview of the emerging role in CCT and CMR for TR patient evaluation, and TTVI planning and follow-up.

CARDIAC COMPUTED TOMOGRAPHY IMAGING ACQUISITION

Patients with TR often have atrial arrhythmias, intracardiac devices, and/or chronic kidney disease which pose challenges for CT imaging. The CT examination for TTVI planning should be performed using CT scanners with either whole-heart single-beat volumetric coverage (up to 16 cm craniocaudal on the z-axis) or dual-source CT scanners with high coverage and temporal resolution.[5] An ECG-gated acquisition covering the whole cardiac cycle, without dose modulation, and using the smallest available collimation (recommended 0.5–0.625 mm) is key for high-quality functional reconstruction (eg, every 5% of the R-R interval). In patients

with arrhythmia and/or high heart rate variability, commonly seen with TR, functional reconstruction in absolute msec increments (eg, every 50 ms, from 0 ms to the duration of the shortest R-R cycle) is advised to mitigate motion and misalignment artifacts for scanners without whole heart, single beat coverage.

The main goal of the contrast injection protocol is to achieve a diagnostic and homogeneous right heart enhancement—ideally greater than 400 Hounsfield Units, without streak artifacts in the superior vena cava or mixing artifacts in the right atrium. Left-sided contrast enhancement is beneficial and often achievable with biphasic injection protocol; it is helpful before transcatheter annuloplasty device planning whereby the right coronary artery relationship to the TA has to be assessed, or for the baseline and follow-up assessment of biventricular function. Contrast infusion requires a dual-head injector and is performed as a bi or triphasic protocol, with variable contrast/saline mixture.[6–8] Depending on BMI and renal function, we use a biphasic contrast injection (80%/20% blend of contrast/saline at 4 mL/s, followed by a 60 mL saline chaser at 3.5 mL/s). Either a bolus tracking technique with the region of interest (ROI) placed at the left atrium (attenuation threshold of 120 HU) or a test bolus method with ROIs in the pulmonary artery and aorta may be applied. Typically, a total contrast volume in the range of 50 to 80 mL is applied for the CT acquisition, depending on patient factors and scanner type. For a comprehensive review of protocols, see Pulerwitz and colleagues.[7]

A delayed nongated helical acquisition of the abdomen and pelvis, typically 50 to 60 seconds after arterial injection, is often obtained to ascertain the venous access size and trajectory necessary for new TTVI replacement devices.

TRICUSPID ANATOMY ESSENTIALS FOR TRANSCATHETER TRICUSPID VALVE INTERVENTIONS
Leaflets and Commissures
The TV leaflets are thinner and are more prone to injury than the mitral valve leaflets. The TV leaflets have a highly variable configuration. The classical 3-leaflet TV is found in 28% to 58% of patients.[9–11] In this configuration, the anterior leaflet is the largest (radially and circumferentially) and most mobile, the septal leaflet is the shortest radially and least mobile, and the posterior leaflet is the shortest circumferentially.[11] In up to one-third of patients, the posterior leaflet is divided by an additional commissure.[11] In rare cases, the TV has only 2-

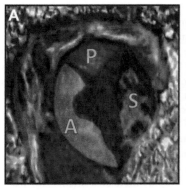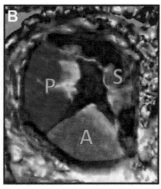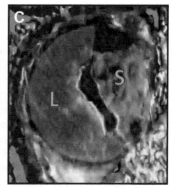

Fig. 2. En-face 3D rendered reconstruction in systolic phase (30%–40%) of the tricuspid valve (TV) leaflets using circle cvi software. (A) Three leaflet TV with a small posterior leaflet (*orange*) and a large anterior leaflet (*green*)—most common anatomy; (B) three leaflet TV with a larger posterior leaflet (*orange*), even larger than the anterior (*green*); (C) bicuspid TV. In addition, the reader can observe the complex shape of the regurgitant orifice in these patients with massive and torrential tricuspid regurgitation. See functional reconstruction in Video 1

leaflets (2%–10% of cases).[9–11] (Fig. 2 and Video 1).

The anteroseptal and posteroseptal coaptation zones of the TV are 2 of the major sites of regurgitation and the target for transcatheter edge-to-edge repair (TEER). Variable scallops and indentations of the posterior and anterior leaflets make the definition of the third (anteroposterior) coaptation line and commissure challenging. Some authors propose the use of the

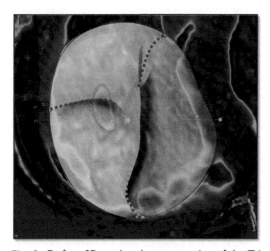

Fig. 3. En-face 3D rendered reconstruction of the TV, with superimposed, transparent leaflet. The three leaflets are shown in pink (septal), blue (anterior), and yellow (posterior); and the three commissures are shown in dotted lines: orange (anteroseptal), red (anteroposterior), and green (posteroseptal). Note the anterior papillary muscle (brown) below the anteroposterior commissure, which serves as an anatomic marker to identify the anteroposterior commissure. See Video 2.

anterior papillary muscle as an anatomic reference to identify the anteroposterior commissure (Fig. 3 and Video 2). Evaluation and delineation of the commissural and leaflet anatomy, coaptation gaps, and chordal attachments are important for TEER procedure planning.

Tricuspid Annulus

The tricuspid annulus (TA) is the largest annulus of the heart. In normal subjects, the average TA diameter is 30 mm and the area 9 cm^2.[12,13] In patients with severe functional TR, the average diameter can reach up to 45 mm and the area can almost double in size (16–17 cm^2).[14,15] In comparison, the mitral valve annulus area averages 12 cm^2 in patients with advanced mitral regurgitation.[16,17]

The TA is very dynamic in normal subjects, with dimensions changing around 20% to 35% through the cardiac cycle. It is largest in late diastole and smallest in mid to late systole. However, this dynamism is often blunted in patients with functional TR.[12,18,19]

Only the septal portion of the TA has fibrous tissue, which is attached to the central fibrous body of the heart and works as a pivot for the hinge-like, systolic excursion of the free wall (or mural) portion of the TA toward the RV apex. The muscle bands that support the annulus follow right chambers contractility. The free wall portions of the TA have little to no fibrous tissue. As such, TA dilation from RV and/or RA enlargement occurs in the direction of the free wall.

The combination of large valve orifice, TA dynamism, and absence of circumferential fibrous support of the TV challenges TR device design and deployment, especially those that depend on annular support for anchoring (eg, replacement devices). However, the large valve orifice permits the implantation of larger coaptation devices (eg, clips) without leading to significant valve stenosis.

Subvalvular Apparatus

Papillary muscles (PM) lend a dense net of chordae to tension the TV leaflets. The anterior PM is typically the largest, with the most constant anatomic characteristics. It attaches to the RV anterior wall, connects to the moderator band, and lends chordal support to the anterior and posterior leaflets. The posterior PM is usually more fragmented, with multiple heads, and lends chordal support to the septal and posterior leaflets. The septal PM, when present, can be single or multiple, and lends fan-shaped chordal support to the septal and anterior leaflets. The septal PM is absent in approximately 20% of patients with the chordae attaching directly to the RV septum.[20,21]

This variable and dense PM network along with accompanying chordal anatomy may affect catheters' and devices' navigation. Simulations and distance measurements to predict potential device interaction with the subvalvular apparatus are important for device-specific TTVI planning.

Adjacent Structures

The evaluation and spatial relationship of adjacent structures to the TV such as the right coronary artery, the His bundle, and the noncoronary sinus of Valsalva (all adjacent to the TV) are important for TTVI planning.

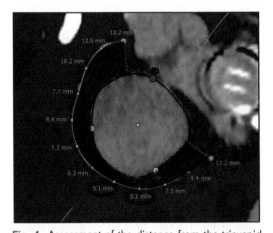

Fig. 4. Assessment of the distance from the tricuspid annulus (TA) to the right coronary artery (RCA) using a dedicated semi-automated tool. Non-coronary cusp (NCC) is in close proximity to the septal-anterior (SA) commissure. The distance is closest between the posterior segment of the TA and the mid-distal transition of the RCA. In this case 5.1 mm.

The right coronary artery courses through the right atrioventricular groove and hugs the anterior and posterior portions of the TA. Iatrogenic injury of the right coronary, although rare, can occur after transcatheter annuloplasty due to its proximity with the TA.[22] The distance to the TA shortens from proximal to distal segments of the right coronary artery, and careful preprocedural CCT assessment is important to identify potential injury (Fig. 4).[23]

The His bundle and the noncoronary sinus of Valsalva are close to the anteroseptal commissure. During deployment and anchoring, transcatheter replacement devices can exert an excessive radial force on this region leading to atrioventricular block or, in extreme cases, aortic perforation at the noncoronary sinus.[20]

CARDIAC COMPUTED TOMOGRAPHY FOR RIGHT-CHAMBER AND TRICUSPID REGURGITATION QUANTIFICATION

Although echocardiography is the main imaging modality for TR severity assessment; functional CCT can provide a complementary assessment of TR severity and right-sided chamber function and remodeling.[4]

Right-sided chambers volumetric and functional assessment is feasible using the same multiphasic, ECG-gated CCT imaging protocol acquisition outlined before. CCT offers the advantage of a 3D, whole-heart volumetric assessment of the complex RV chamber.[24] Fig. 5 and Video 3. The accuracy of RV volumetric and ejection fraction measurements by CCT is comparable to CMR, considered the gold standard of ejection fraction measurement.[25] Proper preprocedural RV assessment is important to ensure that TR reduction will not lead to afterload mismatch, which can worsen right-heart failure. The RV is especially susceptible to pressure overload and TR reduction variably shifts the RV hemodynamic from a volume to a pressure overload environment, depending on the pulmonary pressures, degree of TR reduction, and baseline RV function. Thus, in addition to the anatomic assessment described above, functional evaluation by CCT should be used in preprocedure planning for all patients undergoing TTVI.

Most of the patients with TR have a functional mechanism, with associated TA dilation.[26] The TA size, therefore, correlates with TR severity and can be used as a surrogate marker of TR severity.[4] In addition, functional CCT images can provide the assessment of the TR mechanism and direct measurement of the tricuspid anatomic regurgitant orifice area (AROA). 3D AROA by CCT has a strong correlation with the vena contracta area measured

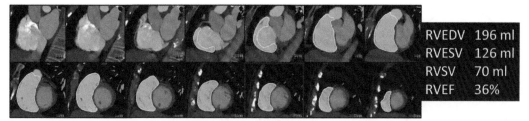

RVEDV	196 ml
RVESV	126 ml
RVSV	70 ml
RVEF	36%

Fig. 5. Right ventricle volumetric assessment using functional CCT reconstructions in the short-axis. See also Video 5.

by 3D TEE,[27] providing an objective assessment of TR severity particularly when echocardiographic images are suboptimal. A detailed, step-by-step approach for the tricuspid AROA measurement is provided in Fig. 6, and additional measurements are detailed in Fig. 7.

CARDIAC COMPUTED TOMOGRAPHY PLANNING FOR PROCEDURAL FLUOROSCOPIC VIEWS

Preprocedural CCT can provide individually tailored optimal fluoroscopic viewing angles for TTVI. In practice, the main procedural viewing angles are the right anterior oblique (RAO) angles for long-axis views of the right-sided chambers, coplanar to the TA, and a caudal left anterior oblique (LAO) angle for a short-axis (en-face) view of the TV, orthogonal to the TA (Fig. 8).[28,29] Specifically, a more caudal RAO angle provides a 2-chamber (or inflow) view and a more cranial RAO angle provides a 3-chamber (or inflow-outflow) view. Both RAO (long-axis) views are used to visualize the delivery system trajectory in the RA to achieve a co-axial approach to the TV. The more caudal RAO view (2-chamber), with the inferior vena cava in-plane, is used to visualize the delivery

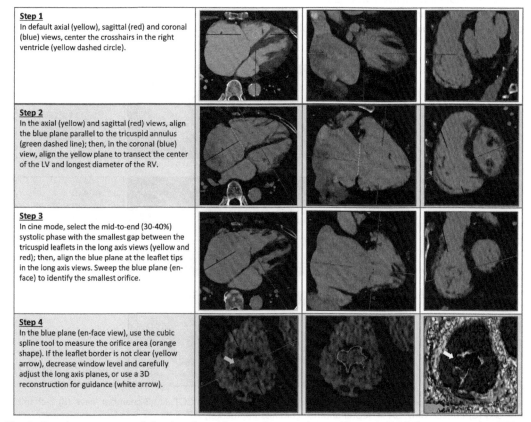

Fig. 6. Step-by-step approach for the tricuspid anatomic regurgitant orifice area (AROA) assessment by CCT.

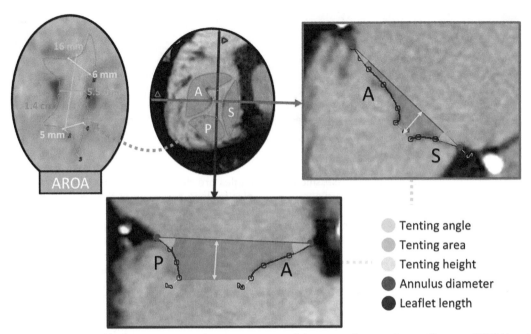

Fig. 7. Assessment of leaflet anatomy, tenting parameters, and the anatomic regurgitant orifice area (AROA) and coaptation gaps.

system advancing through the vena cava and the RA, and the more cranial RAO view (3-chamber) to adjust coaxiality and orientation (anterior vs posterior) of the delivery system since its plane is aligned to the coaptation line of the septal leaflet with the anterior and posterior leaflets. The short-axis view is used to visualize the delivery system steering and alignment of device

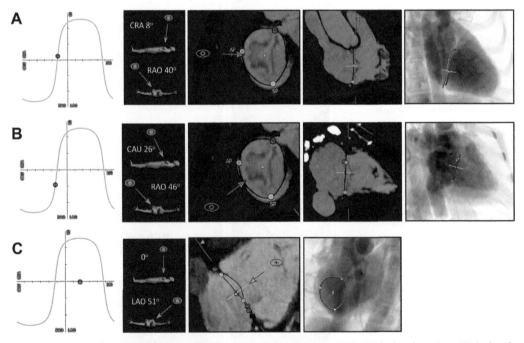

Fig. 8. Pre-procedural prediction of the main fluoroscopic angles using CCT. (A) 3-chamber view, (B) 2-chamber view, and (C) en-face view. SA = septal-anterior commissural marker; AP, antero-posterior commissural marker; SP, septal-posterior commissural marker.

parts (eg, clips arms) to the target (eg, perpendicular to the coaptation plane); during annuloplasty device anchoring, it can also be used to monitor the right coronary artery proximity, avoiding injury, and/or spasm.

CARDIAC COMPUTED TOMOGRAPHY PLANNING FOR TRANSCATHETER TRICUSPID VALVE INTERVENTIONS ACCORDING TO THE DEVICE TYPE

Several TTVI devices that mimic surgical approaches are under investigation in early feasibility and randomized clinical trials. Based on their mechanisms of TR reduction, these devices can be classified into 4 categories: TEER devices, annuloplasty devices, replacement devices, and heterotopic caval devices. Each device type requires a specific preprocedural imaging protocol and analysis, most of which have a central CCT component. In-depth imaging protocols for each, constantly evolving, devices are beyond the scope of this review; however, the following section provides an overview of the essential measurements for the most currently investigated devices.

EDGE-TO-EDGE REPAIR COAPTATION DEVICES

TEER reduces TR via approximation of the tricuspid leaflets, mimicking Alfieri's surgical repair. The TriClip device (Abbott Vascular, Santa Clara, CA) restores leaflet coaptation by clipping and approximating leaflets' edges in a similar fashion to the MitraClip (Abbott Vascular, Santa Clara, CA), but with a different delivery system, optimized for the TV. The PASCAL device (Edwards Lifesciences, Irvine, CA) has 2 paddles and clasps, which attach to the leaflets' edges and approximates it to a central spacer that fills the gap between leaflets.

For TEER devices, echocardiography is the main imaging modality for patient selection and preprocedural planning, and patients without adequate acoustic windows on TEE are usually excluded from these treatments. Functional CCT, although not routinely performed for TEER, may provide morphological and functional characterization of the TV and TR mechanism. This includes leaflet mobility, leaflet length, leaflet tenting, coaptation gaps, and leaflet interaction with pacemaker and defibrillator leads (see **Fig. 7** and Video 4). CCT can also simulate the delivery catheter trajectory to anticipate steering difficulties (**Fig. 9**).

ANNULOPLASTY DEVICES

Transcatheter annuloplasty devices (eg, Cardioband [Edwards Lifesciences, Irvine, CA, USA] and Millipede [Boston Scientific, Marlborough, MA, USA]) emulate surgical annuloplasty. Annuloplasty devices require preprocedural CCT to assess: TA dimensions throughout the cardiac cycle for device size selection (**Fig. 10** and Video 4), anatomic landmarks (eg, leaflets commissures, tissue quality around the TA, and proximity to the right coronary artery) to define the ideal positioning of anchors (**Fig. 11**), potential right atrial wall contact, and optimal fluoroscopic projection (see **Fig. 8**).[30,31] In patients with functional TR, the tenting height obtained from CCT may be useful to predict the risk of TR recurrence after annuloplasty.[32] Each device has specific measurements and planning which go beyond the scope of this review.

REPLACEMENT DEVICES

Transcatheter tricuspid valve replacement (TTVR) devices are in early feasibility trials and are typically considered for patients with unsuitable anatomy for TEER (highly retracted septal leaflet, large coaptation gaps (>10 mm), or tenting height (>7–10 mm), commonly observed in those with torrential TR grades). Several TTVR devices are available with varying sizes and delivery systems. Preprocedural CCT planning identifies anatomic characteristics and device suitability. Annulus sizing and virtual valve simulation using preprocedural CCT images are important steps for device selection **Fig. 12**. One of the main barriers, given late presentation and evaluation of these patients has been significantly dilated TA which becomes an exclusion criterion for currently available TTVR devices. For example, the largest devices available are the 48 mm Intrepid device (Medtronic, Mounds View, MN), the 52 mm EVOQUE (Edwards Lifesciences, Irvine, CA, USA), and the 55 mm cardiovalve (Boston Medical, Shrewsbury, MA, USA). TTVR delivery systems vary in size from 28Fr to 42Fr, and venous access must be measured typically on a delayed acquisition approximately 50 seconds after the arterial phase to assess the sheath/femoral vein ratio. Measurements of superior and inferior vena cava should be taken, in addition to their relationship to the TA to ensure adequate navigation of the delivery system. Individual anatomy varies (especially in the instance of right chamber remodeling) and preprocedural CCT simulation can help to predict delivery system trajectory and intraprocedural steering difficulties.[33];

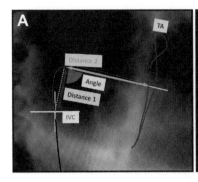
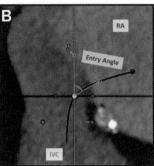

Fig. 9. Catheter simulation for TTVI. After tracing the inferior vena cavae (*yellow*) orifice and tricuspid annulus (red), a cubic spline trajectory connecting the center of both structures in a coaxial manner is estimated for the catheter (*dark blue*). (*A*) The distances from the IVC to the TA central, coaxial plane (distance 1) and the distance from the intersection of the central, coaxial planes to the TA (distance 2) is provided, as well as the angle of intersection of both planes. (*B*) It is also possible to evaluate the angle from the IVC to the central, coaxial plane of the TA.

CAVAL HETEROTOPIC DEVICES

Caval heterotopic devices are typically indicated as a palliative option for patients ineligible for TTVI due to anatomic and/or functional. In this procedure, a stented valve is implanted in either the inferior vena cava or both the inferior and superior vena cava to reduce the reflux from the RA to the vena cava. It may relieve systemic venous congestion and hepatic dysfunction, but it does not improve TR severity because it does not halt right-sided chamber remodeling.

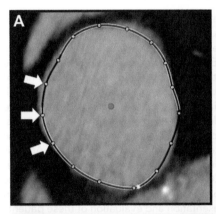
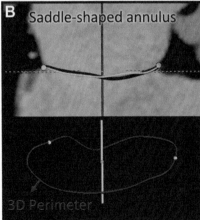
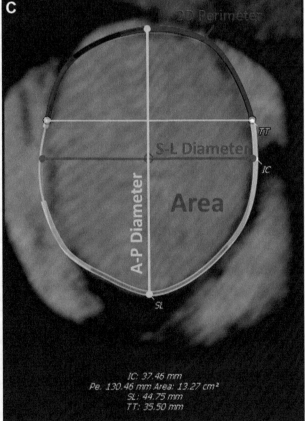

Fig. 10. For the tricuspid annulus (TA) sizing, we manually place 16 markers on the hinge points where leaflets connect to the TA (*A, white arrows*), and it automatically generates a 3D model using cubic spline interpolation which accounts for its nonplanar, saddle-shaped TA morphology (*B*). The tracings are performed in end-systolic and end-diastolic phases of the cardiac cycle. (*C*) 4 parameters are measured: perimeter (2D and 3D), area, anteroposterior (A-P) diameter and septal-lateral diameter.

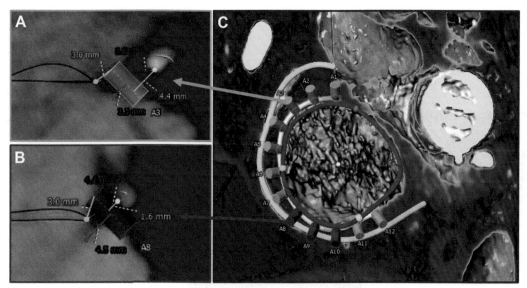

Fig. 11. Simulation of the Cardioband anchors positioning (*C*) and evaluation of its proximity to the right coronary artery on CCT images. Anchors in blue have a safe distance from the right coronary artery (*A*) and anchors in red have are closer to the annulus (*B*) implying an increased risk of coronary injury.

Two devices were designed for this purpose—the Tricento (New Valve Technology, Hechingen, Germany) and the TricValve (P & F Products & Features Vertriebs GmbH, Vienna, Austria). The latter is being studied in an ongoing early feasibility trial (TRICUS [NCT03723239]). Preprocedural CCT is routinely performed to measure the diameters of the inferior and the superior vena cava for device sizing and evaluation of the landing zone to avoid hepatic vein occlusion **Fig. 13**.

CARDIAC MAGNETIC RESONANCE FOR THE EVALUATION OF RIGHT VENTRICULAR SIZE AND FUNCTION

CMR has the advantage of assessing cardiac anatomy and function with high spatial resolution without ionizing radiation or contrast injection while not being limited to the body habitus and/or echocardiographic windows. CMR is currently the gold standard for assessing RV morphology and systolic function, and dedicated RV views from multiple planes allow for a comprehensive assessment of the complex RV anatomy and morphology. Multiple challenges for CMR acquisition in these patients are related to the frequent presence of atrial fibrillation (>80% of patients being considered for TTVI), presence of intracardiac devices such as pacemakers or ICDs, and often inability to perform breath-hold. Several technological CMR developments have become available over the last 5 years which have allowed for single-breath hold[34] or complete free-breathing imaging

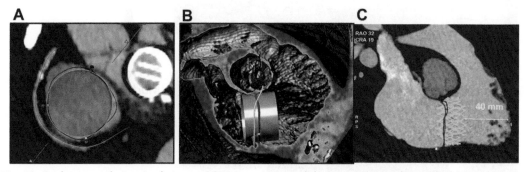

Fig. 12. Replacement device simulation on CCT image. (*A*) Virtual device sizing according to the tricuspid annulus measurement. (*B*) 3D rendered reconstruction showing the virtual device and its relationship with surrounding structures including the subvalvular apparatus and right ventricle output tract. (*C*) Stereolithography of TTVI device (48 mm Intrepid, Medtronic) simulated and distance from device to the RV border.

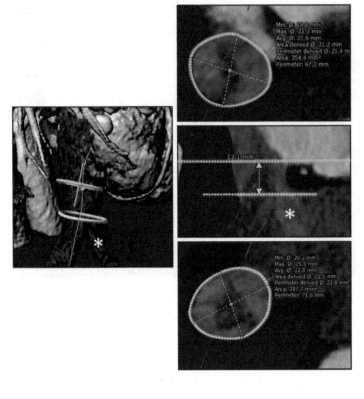

Fig. 13. Preprocedural measurements of the inferior vena cava (IVC) for caval heterotopic device sizing and positioning. After the IVC centerline is traced, 2 transverse planes are defined, the transition plane from the IVC to the right atrium (*blue*) and at the level of the first hepatic vein (*yellow*). Measurements of the IVC size (area, diameters and perimeter) and the distance between the planes are provided.

acquisition,[35] in the most vulnerable patients with atrial arrhythmias.[36]

CARDIAC MAGNETIC RESONANCE FOR TRICUSPID REGURGITATION QUANTIFICATION

CMR assessment of TR is less established than that of other regurgitant valvular diseases.

However, CMR can quantify TR volume and TR fraction by direct (subtracting the LV from the RV stroke volume) and more commonly by the indirect method (subtracting the flow through the pulmonary artery [obtained from phase-contrast imaging] from RV stroke volume [obtained from RV 3D volumetric analysis]). In addition to the ability to assess right-sided-chamber remodeling and function, CMR can

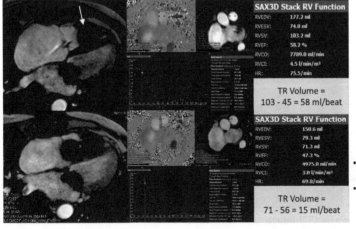

Fig. 14. TTVI CMR evaluation in a patient with prior pacemaker, who underwent leadless pacemaker implantation (white arrow) with residual significant TR quantified by CMR. Patient underwent TTVI using TEER device (TriClip, Abbott Structural) with significant improvement of TR 1 month after TTVI.

RV and LV infarct seen on delayed enhancement imaging

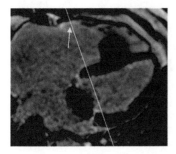 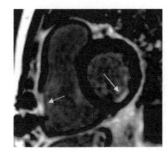

Fig. 15. TTVI CMR evaluation on the same patient as Fig. 14, with late gadolinium enhancement imaging showing small subendocardial infarction involving the basal anterior RV free-wall and basal inferior LV consistent with prior right coronary artery infarct (yellow arrow).

play a complementary role to echocardiography in TR severity assessment which can be important for decision making and timing of intervention. Echocardiographic assessment of TR severity requires many parameters which are not hierarchically oriented leading to a moderate diagnostic concordance rate of 65% between echocardiography and CMR.[37]

Quantitative evaluation of TR by CMR was associated with mortality in a recent study of 547 patients with significant functional TR.[38] A TR volume ≥45 mL or a TR fraction ≥50% was associated with increased mortality at 5-years follow-up. However, this cohort excluded patients with atrial fibrillation or implantable devices at the time of imaging because of inherent beat-to-beat variability in TR and metal artifacts, which limits the generalizability of these findings.

POSTTRANSCATHETER TRICUSPID VALVE INTERVENTION IMAGING EVALUATION
Tricuspid regurgitation reduction
The pre- and post-TTVI CMR imaging is shown for a patient with severe TR (Fig. 14). The TR volume was calculated using the indirect method (subtracting the flow through the pulmonary artery from the RV stroke volume). In this case, there was a coexistence of a leadless pacemaker in the right ventricular apex and chronic atrial fibrillation. Although the quantification of the right ventricular volume was partially limited due to artifacts, TR severity evaluation was still feasible. Three-months postprocedure the TR fraction reduced from 56% to 21% with an increase in RV forward flow. Despite the imaging obstacles due to the aforementioned artifacts, the CMR potential to evaluate interval response of TTVI treatment is currently under development for patients with severe TR.[39,40]

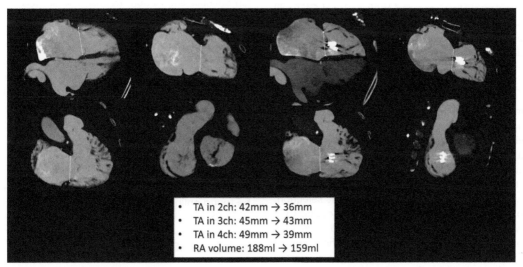

- TA in 2ch: 42mm → 36mm
- TA in 3ch: 45mm → 43mm
- TA in 4ch: 49mm → 39mm
- RA volume: 188ml → 159ml

Fig. 16. CCT evaluation pre- and post-TEER demonstrating TA annular changes after leaflet therapy. RA and RV volumes also decreased 1 month after TTVI.

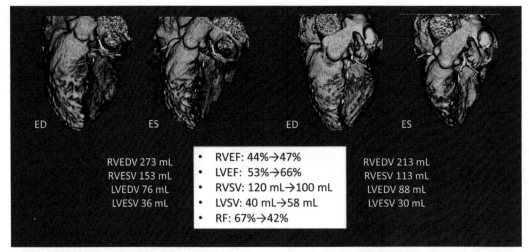

- RVEDV 273 mL
- RVESV 153 mL
- LVEDV 76 mL
- LVESV 36 mL

- RVEF: 44%→47%
- LVEF: 53%→66%
- RVSV: 120 mL→100 mL
- LVSV: 40 mL→58 mL
- RF: 67%→42%

- RVEDV 213 mL
- RVESV 113 mL
- LVEDV 88 mL
- LVESV 30 mL

Fig. 17. Functional CCT 3D reconstruction pre- and post-TEER (TriClip, Abbott Structural). Note the reverse remodeling and improvement of biventricular systolic functional 1 month after TEER.

CMR can additionally detect RV and LV myocardial fibrosis by late gadolinium enhancement or extracellular volume quantification (**Fig. 15**). In left-sided valvular heart diseases, myocardial fibrosis quantified by CMR is associated with pathologic left ventricular remodeling and mortality.[41,42] Further research is necessary to understand the prognostic impact of RV myocardial fibrosis in patients with TR, although we acknowledge the challenges of tissue characterization of the thin-walled RV.

Reverse remodeling

Multiphasic CCT can assess right-sided chambers reverse remodeling after TTVI. CCT can quantify changes in the TA, RV volumes, and RVEF[43] (**Fig. 16** and **17**). Many of the quantitative parameters assessed by functional CCT will be evaluated in future trials which will require post-TTVI imaging by regulatory agencies to understand device performance.

SUMMARY

In this rapidly evolving field of TTVI, advanced imaging modalities such as CCT and CMR will provide an important contribution to the complex anatomic and functional assessment of the RV structure, size, function, and quantification of TR severity. Together, this incremental information will be used to better inform patient selection, plan, guide, and assess procedural results. CCT which has been already an integral part of TTVI planning is well suited to evaluate the complex 3D functional and anatomic changes occurring on the right side after interventions. CMR, the gold standard for morphologic and functional assessment of the RV, is a reproducible method for TR quantification, although less available and explored in this challenging population, it has potential applications on the understanding of the RV remodeling and functional recovery, and TR reduction post-TTVI. The success of TTVI will remain highly dependent on a well-integrated heart team encompassing heart surgeons, interventional cardiologists, and cardiac imagers with advanced imaging expertise to understand the strengths and complementary applications of the different imaging modalities for these patients.

DISCLOSURE

J.L. Cavalcante has received consulting fees from Boston Scientific and Abbott Vascular; and has received research grant support from Circle Cardiovascular Imaging, Edwards Lifesciences, Medtronic, Boston Scientific, and Abbott Vascular. P. Sorajja has received consulting fees from Abbott Structural, Medtronic, Boston Scientific, Edwards Lifesciences, Gore, and Teleflex; and has received research grant support from Abbott Structural, Medtronic, and Boston Scientific. V.N. Bapat has received consulting fees from Medtronic, Edwards Lifesciences, Abbott Structural, Boston Scientific, 4C.

SUPPLEMENTARY DATA

Supplementary data related to this article can be found online at https://doi.org/10.1016/j.iccl.2021.09.004.

REFERENCES

1. Zack CJ, Fender EA, Chandrashekar P, et al. National Trends and Outcomes in Isolated Tricuspid

Valve Surgery. J Am Coll Cardiol 2017;70(24):2953–60.

2. Asmarats L, Puri R, Latib A, et al. Transcatheter Tricuspid Valve Interventions: Landscape, Challenges, and Future Directions. J Am Coll Cardiol 2018;71(25):2935–56.

3. Agricola E, Asmarats L, Maisano F, et al. Imaging for Tricuspid Valve Repair and Replacement. JACC Cardiovasc Imaging 2020. https://doi.org/10.1016/j.jcmg.2020.01.031. S1936878X20305374.

4. Hahn RT, Thomas JD, Khalique OK, et al. Imaging Assessment of Tricuspid Regurgitation Severity. JACC Cardiovasc Imaging 2019;12(3):469–90.

5. Lewis MA, Pascoal A, Keevil SF, et al. Selecting a CT scanner for cardiac imaging: the heart of the matter. Br J Radiol 2016;89(1065):20160376.

6. van Rosendael PJ, Kamperidis V, Kong WKF, et al. Computed tomography for planning transcatheter tricuspid valve therapy. Eur Heart J 2017;38(9):665–74.

7. Pulerwitz TC, Khalique OK, Leb J, et al. Optimizing Cardiac CT Protocols for Comprehensive Acquisition Prior to Percutaneous MV and TV Repair/Replacement. JACC Cardiovasc Imaging 2019. https://doi.org/10.1016/j.jcmg.2019.01.041.

8. Saremi F, Hassani C, Millan-Nunez V, et al. Imaging Evaluation of Tricuspid Valve: Analysis of Morphology and Function With CT and MRI. AJR Am J Roentgenol 2015;204(5):W531–42.

9. Wafae N, Hayashi H, Gerola LR, et al. Anatomical study of the human tricuspid valve. Surg Radiol Anat SRA 1990;12(1):37–41.

10. Hołda MK, Zhingre Sanchez JD, Bateman MG, et al. Right Atrioventricular Valve Leaflet Morphology Redefined: Implications for Transcatheter Repair Procedures. JACC Cardiovasc Interv 2019;12(2):169–78.

11. Hahn RT, Weckbach LT, Noack T, et al. Proposal for a standard echocardiographic tricuspid valve Nomenclature. JACC Cardiovasc imaging 2021. https://doi.org/10.1016/j.jcmg.2021.01.012. S1936878X21000759.

12. Addetia K, Muraru D, Veronesi F, et al. 3-Dimensional Echocardiographic Analysis of the Tricuspid Annulus Provides New Insights Into Tricuspid Valve Geometry and Dynamics. JACC Cardiovasc Imaging 2019;12(3):401–12.

13. Zhan Y, Debs D, Khan MA, et al. Normal Reference Values and Reproducibility of Tricuspid Annulus Dimensions Using Cardiovascular Magnetic Resonance. Am J Cardiol 2019;124(4):594–8.

14. Praz F, Khalique OK, Dos Reis Macedo LG, et al. Comparison between Three-Dimensional Echocardiography and Computed Tomography for Comprehensive Tricuspid Annulus and Valve Assessment in Severe Tricuspid Regurgitation: Implications for Tricuspid Regurgitation Grading and

Transcatheter Therapies. J Am Soc Echocardiogr Off Publ Am Soc Echocardiogr 2018;31(11):1190–202. e3.

15. van Rosendael PJ, Joyce E, Katsanos S, et al. Tricuspid valve remodelling in functional tricuspid regurgitation: multidetector row computed tomography insights. Eur Heart J Cardiovasc Imaging 2016;17(1):96–105.

16. Tang Z, Fan Y-T, Wang Y, et al. Mitral Annular and Left Ventricular Dynamics in Atrial Functional Mitral Regurgitation: A Three-Dimensional and Speckle-Tracking Echocardiographic Study. J Am Soc Echocardiogr Off Publ Am Soc Echocardiogr 2019;32(4):503–13.

17. Naoum C, Leipsic J, Cheung A, et al. Mitral Annular Dimensions and Geometry in Patients With Functional Mitral Regurgitation and Mitral Valve Prolapse: Implications for Transcatheter Mitral Valve Implantation. JACC Cardiovasc Imaging 2016;9(3):269–80.

18. Maffessanti F, Gripari P, Pontone G, et al. Three-dimensional dynamic assessment of tricuspid and mitral annuli using cardiovascular magnetic resonance. Eur Heart J Cardiovasc Imaging 2013;14(10):986–95.

19. Ring L, Rana BS, Kydd A, et al. Dynamics of the tricuspid valve annulus in normal and dilated right hearts: a three-dimensional transoesophageal echocardiography study. Eur Heart J Cardiovasc Imaging 2012;13(9):756–62.

20. Dahou A, Levin D, Reisman M, et al. Anatomy and Physiology of the Tricuspid Valve. JACC Cardiovasc Imaging 2019;12(3):458–68.

21. Faletra FF, Leo LA, Paiocchi VL, et al. Imaging-based tricuspid valve anatomy by computed tomography, magnetic resonance imaging, two and three-dimensional echocardiography: correlation with anatomic specimen. Eur Heart J Cardiovasc Imaging 2019;20(1):1–13.

22. Vollroth M, Sandri M, Garbade J, et al. Severe right coronary artery injury during minimally invasive tricuspid valve repair. Eur J Cardio-thorac Surg Off J Eur Assoc Cardio-thorac Surg 2015;48(3):e62.

23. Hinzpeter R, Eberhard M, Pozzoli A, et al. Dynamic anatomic relationship of coronary arteries to the valves. Part 2: tricuspid annulus and right coronary artery. Eurointervention J Eur Collab Work Group Interv Cardiol Eur Soc Cardiol 2019;15(10):935–8.

24. Karam N, Mehr M, Taramasso M, et al. Value of Echocardiographic Right Ventricular and Pulmonary Pressure Assessment in Predicting Transcatheter Tricuspid Repair Outcome. JACC Cardiovasc Interv 2020. https://doi.org/10.1016/j.jcin.2020.02.028.

25. Maffei E, Messalli G, Martini C, et al. Left and right ventricle assessment with Cardiac CT: validation study vs. Cardiac MR. Eur Radiol 2012;22(5):1041–9.

26. Ton-Nu T-T, Levine RA, Handschumacher MD, et al. Geometric determinants of functional tricuspid regurgitation: insights from 3-dimensional echocardiography. Circulation 2006;114(2):143–9.

27. Lopes BBC, Sorajja P, Hashimoto G, et al. Tricuspid Anatomic Regurgitant Orifice Area by Functional DSCT: A Novel Parameter of Tricuspid Regurgitation Severity. JACC Cardiovasc Imaging. Published online March 10, 2021. doi:10.1016/j.jcmg.2021.02.002

28. Pighi M, Thériault-Lauzier P, Alosaimi H, et al. Fluoroscopic Anatomy of Right-Sided Heart Structures for Transcatheter Interventions. JACC Cardiovasc Interv 2018;11(16):1614–25.

29. Pozzoli A, Maisano F, Kuwata S, et al. Fluoroscopic anatomy of the tricuspid valve: Implications for Transcatheter procedures. Int J Cardiol 2017;244:119–20.

30. Mangieri A, Lim S, Rogers JH, et al. Percutaneous Tricuspid Annuloplasty. Interv Cardiol Clin 2018;7(1):31–6.

31. Wunderlich NC, Landendinger M, Arnold M, et al. State-of-the-Art Review: Anatomical and Imaging Considerations During Transcatheter Tricuspid Valve Repair Using an Annuloplasty Approach. Front Cardiovasc Med 2021;8:619605.

32. Kabasawa M, Kohno H, Ishizaka T, et al. Assessment of functional tricuspid regurgitation using 320-detector-row multislice computed tomography: risk factor analysis for recurrent regurgitation after tricuspid annuloplasty. J Thorac Cardiovasc Surg 2014;147(1):312–20.

33. Hahn RT. State-of-the-Art Review of Echocardiographic Imaging in the Evaluation and Treatment of Functional Tricuspid Regurgitation. Circ Cardiovasc Imaging 2016;9(12). https://doi.org/10.1161/CIRCIMAGING.116.005332.

34. Vermersch M, Longère B, Coisne A, et al. Compressed sensing real-time cine imaging for assessment of ventricular function, volumes and mass in clinical practice. Eur Radiol 2020;30(1):609–19.

35. Merlocco A, Olivieri L, Kellman P, et al. Improved Workflow for Quantification of Right Ventricular Volumes Using Free-Breathing Motion Corrected Cine Imaging. Pediatr Cardiol 2019;40(1):79–88.

36. Wang J, Lin Q, Pan Y, et al. The accuracy of compressed sensing cardiovascular magnetic resonance imaging in heart failure classifications. Int J Cardiovasc Imaging 2020;36(6):1157–66.

37. Zhan Y, Senapati A, Vejpongsa P, et al. Comparison of Echocardiographic Assessment of Tricuspid Regurgitation Against Cardiovascular Magnetic Resonance. JACC Cardiovasc Imaging 2020;13(7):1461–71.

38. Zhan Y, Debs D, Khan MA, et al. Natural History of Functional Tricuspid Regurgitation Quantified by Cardiovascular Magnetic Resonance. J Am Coll Cardiol 2020;76(11):1291–301.

39. Rommel K-P, Besler C, Noack T, et al. Physiological and Clinical Consequences of Right Ventricular Volume Overload Reduction After Transcatheter Treatment for Tricuspid Regurgitation. JACC Cardiovasc Interv 2019;12(15):1423–34.

40. Hashimoto G, Fukui M, Sorajja P, et al. Essential roles for CT and MRI in timing of therapy in tricuspid regurgitation. Prog Cardiovasc Dis Published Online December 2019. https://doi.org/10.1016/j.pcad.2019.11.018. S0033062019301598.

41. Puls M, Beuthner BE, Topci R, et al. Impact of myocardial fibrosis on left ventricular remodelling, recovery, and outcome after transcatheter aortic valve implantation in different haemodynamic subtypes of severe aortic stenosis. Eur Heart J 2020;41(20):1903–14.

42. Cavalcante JL, Kusunose K, Obuchowski NA, et al. Prognostic impact of ischemic mitral regurgitation severity and myocardial infarct quantification by cardiovascular magnetic resonance. JACC Cardiovasc Imaging 2020;13(7):1489–501. https://doi.org/10.1016/j.jcmg.2019.11.008.

43. Bc Lopes B, Sorajja P, Hashimoto G, et al. Early Effects of Transcatheter Edge-to-Edge Leaflet Repair for Tricuspid Regurgitation: First-in-Human Experience with Computed Tomography. J Cardiovasc Comput Tomogr 2021;15(2):e12–4. https://doi.org/10.1016/j.jcct.2020.10.001.

Surgical Correction of Tricuspid Regurgitation

Amalia A. Jonsson, MD*, Michael E. Halkos, MD, MSc

KEYWORDS

• Tricuspid annuloplasty • Tricuspid regurgitation • Tricuspid ring • Tricuspid anatomy

---

KEY POINTS

• The tricuspid valve is a complex functional unit comprised of the annulus, leaflets, right atrium, and right ventricle.
• The annular dilation seen in TR is not symmetric, and an annuloplasty needs to restore normal geometry.
• In patients undergoing repair of a degenerative mitral valve, the question of how to treat tricuspid regurgitation is a subject of debate.
• The tricuspid valve is an often forgotten but relevant cause of significant morbidity and mortality.

 Video content accompanies this article at http://www.interventional.theclinics.com.

INTRODUCTION

• Tricuspid anatomy is complex due to its dynamic saddle shape and variable leaflet morphology making it a challenge to repair.
• The most common cause of TR is annular dilation which is asymmetric, primarily affecting the posterior leaflet.
• Tricuspid valve operations remain moderately high risk, with 30-day mortality around 6% to 9%. Reoperation for recurrent TR has a high mortality and carries a 35% 30-day mortality.

Historically opinions on the management of tricuspid regurgitation have been inconsistent. Early methods for handing an incompetent tricuspid valve involved a suture annuloplasty as described by DeVega in 1972 or a commissuroplasty in which a 2 leaflet valve is created as described by Kay in 1974. Valves that could not be repaired required replacement. The prosthetic valves available at the time were first-generation mechanical valves that had a high rate of thrombotic complications. In his 1974, paper Carpentier described a 31% mortality for patients undergoing mitral and tricuspid replacement, and 40% for patients having both valves repaired.[1] At the time, equally acceptable results were demonstrated for tricuspid repair and replacement, as well as conservative management where the tricuspid was not intervened on, and this high mortality was attributed to advanced underlying disease processes.[1]

It is estimated that 1.6 million Americans have moderate to severe TR; however, tricuspid valve procedures are relatively uncommon representing only 3% of cardiac surgeries performed today.[2,3] Patients with severe TR present with predominantly right-sided heart failure symptoms. Initial medical therapy includes lifestyle modifications and diuretics or in the case of secondary TR, treatment of the underlying cause with pulmonary vasodilators for pulmonary hypertension or medical therapy for left ventricular dysfunction. Tricuspid regurgitation is a cause of major morbidity and mortality. Mortality increases with increasing TR severity, even in the absence of ventricular dysfunction or pulmonary hypertension.[4] For patients with heart failure, 1-year survival

---

Division of Cardiothoracic Surgery, Department of Surgery, Emory University School of Medicine, Atlanta, GA, USA
* Corresponding author. Emory Saint Joseph's Hospital, 5665 Peachtree Dunwoody Road Harisson Pavillion, Suite 200, Atlanta, GA 30342.
E-mail address: amalia.jonsson@emory.edu

Intervent Cardiol Clin 11 (2022) 41–50
https://doi.org/10.1016/j.iccl.2021.09.007
2211-7458/22/© 2021 Elsevier Inc. All rights reserved.

declines significantly with increasing TR from 73.4% and 65.9% to 58.7% for none to mild, moderate, and severe respectively,[5] and at 9 years is significantly lower at 43% versus 63% for those without significant TR.[6]

SURGICAL ANATOMY

The tricuspid valve is a complex functional unit comprised of the annulus, leaflets, right atrium, and right ventricle (Fig. 1). The tricuspid annulus is comprised of fibrotic and elastic fibers, located deep to the junction of the leaflet and the right atrium. The anatomic structures at risk during tricuspid surgery include the conduction system and the aortic valve and right coronary artery. The AV node is located within the triangle of Koch, which is defined by the septal leaflet, the tendon of Todaro, and the opening of the coronary sinus. The bundle of His is found at the apex of the triangle, near the anteroseptal

commissure. The aortic valve, specifically the commissure between the non and right coronary sinuses, is also at risk during tricuspid valve surgery as it is separated by only a few millimeters from the tricuspid annulus.

The tricuspid valve annulus has a dynamic saddle shape with the anteroseptal commissure and the posteroseptal commissure being the lowest points. The annular attachment of the anterior leaflet is the highest. The annulus changes shape during the cardiac cycle as the ventricles contract, the aortic root bulges into the anterior annulus, and the posterior annulus folds in toward the septal annulus.

Although described as having 3 separate leaflets, from the surgeons' view this can be a challenge to delineate. The posterior leaflet can have a variable number of cusps making the appearance of the posteroseptal commissure not immediately apparent; however, the true leaflet identity can be found by identifying the

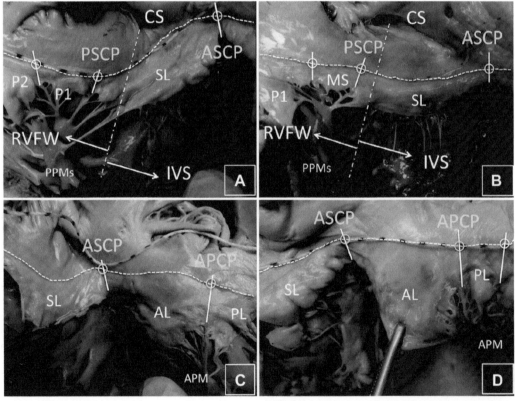

Fig. 1. Leaflet anatomy. Pictures A and B show how the posteroseptal commissure (PSC) can be difficult to identify. Picture B shows a mini scallop (MS) of the posterior leaflet (PL) which can obscure the surgeons' understanding of the anatomy. If the folding point of the right ventricular free wall (RVFW) indicated by the dashed line cannot be identified, the coronary sinus (CS) may help identify its location. Pictures C and D show the relatively uniform shape of the anterior leaflet (AL) which makes it easy to distinguish. APCP, anteroposterior commissural point; APM, anterior papillary muscle; ASCP, anteroseptal commissural point; IVS, interventricular septum; PPM, posterior papillary muscle; PSCP, posteroseptal commissural point SL, septal leaflet.[7]

ventricular attachments (**Fig. 2**). The septal leaflet is supported by the interventricular septum, attached by a fan of chordae inserting directly into the muscle. A small portion of the septal leaflet annulus overhangs the right ventricular free wall in many cadavers.[7] The anterior leaflet is supported by the supraventricular crest, and the entirety of the posterior leaflet annulus is located on the right ventricular free wall. Misjudgment of the location of the posteroseptal commissure can lead to an incorrectly positioned band or ring causing inadequate annular compression and can occur when a prominent scallop is present in the posterior leaflet resulting in a ring that does not extend to the septal portion of the annulus.

Understanding this anatomy is crucial to restoring a competent valve. The asymmetric dilation seen in tricuspid regurgitation results because the geometry of the interventricular septum does not change as the right ventricular size increases compared with the ventricular free wall and to a lesser degree, the supraventricular crest, which have the ability to dilate resulting in leaflet tethering and loss of coaptation. Annuloplasty, therefore, needs to focus on compressing this segment of the annulus primarily.

TRICUSPID VALVE DYSFUNCTION

Tricuspid valve disease can be classified into primary TR or secondary TR. In primary TR, the regurgitation is due to pathology within the tricuspid valve, this can be iatrogenic from pacemaker leads, acquired due to rheumatic tricuspid valve disease, endocarditis, or carcinoid disease, or congenital such as is seen in Ebstein anomaly. It can also occur because of leaflet prolapse as is typically seen with primary mitral regurgitation. In secondary, or functional, TR the tricuspid dysfunction is a result of dysfunction of the left or right ventricle, aortic, or mitral valve disease, or elevated pulmonary artery pressures.

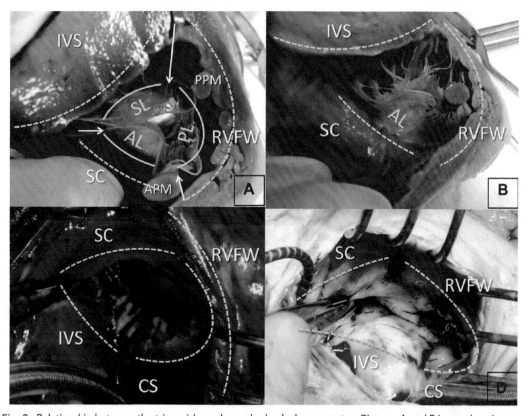

Fig. 2. Relationship between the tricuspid annulus and subvalvular apparatus. Pictures A and B in a cadaveric specimen show much of the septal leaflet (SL) originating from the interventricular septum (IVS), with a part of this leaflet connecting to the right ventricular free wall (RVFW). The posterior leaflet (PL) originates from the RVFW. Most of the anterior leaflet (AL) annulus is supported by the supraventricular crest (SC). Pictures C and D show an intraoperative view of the folding point on the septal leaflet (SL) toward the RVFW, as well as that on the anterior wall from the SC to the RVFW. PPM-posterior papillary muscle, APM-anterior papillary muscle, CS-coronary sinus.[7]

Carpentier functional classification can be applied to regurgitant tricuspid valves similarly as it is to mitral valves. Type I for which the leaflet motion is normal is usually the result of annular dilation. Type II for which the regurgitation occurs due to excess leaflet motion can occur due to ruptured or elongated chordae, or leaflet destruction. Type II disease is most commonly caused by endocarditis, trauma, or iatrogenic causes (intracardiac leads). Type IIIa is typically seen in rheumatic disease and is characterized by restricted leaflet motion in diastole; however, in the cases of rheumatic valves, restriction can also occur in systole. Type IIIb disease is due to ventricular dilation causing leaflet tethering and restricted motion in systole. The most common cause of tricuspid regurgitation in the developing world is mitral valve disease though elevated pulmonary arterial pressures leading to elevated right ventricular pressures, or a dilated right ventricle causing increased tension on the chordae and TV tethering.[8] Other common causes include atrial fibrillation, pacemaker leads, right heart enlargement.

Understanding the geometry of the tricuspid valve is important for successful valvuloplasty. In the case of annular dilation, not all of the leaflets are affected equally. The posterior leaflet is the most severely affected and can increase up to 80% of its annular length. The anterior leaflet can see a 40% increase in length, and the septal leaflet, which is largely unaffected due to its attachment to the interventricular septum, sees only a 10% increase[1] (**Fig. 3**). This asymmetric dilation can be demonstrated on echocardiography. Functionally regurgitant valves have anteroposterior diameters of 48.30 mm ± 6.12 mm which is an 88% increase from normal valves with an AP diameter of 25.59 mm ± 3.2 mm. The medial to lateral distance increases only 31% from 33.71 mm ± 4.52 mm. Additionally, as the annulus dilates it also loses its saddle shape and becomes flat. The height from highest to lowest point of a functionally normal tricuspid valve is 7.23 mm ± 1.05 mm. In

comparison, a functionally regurgitant valve has a height of 4.14 mm ± 1.05 mm.[9] By altering this planar geometry, leaflet tethering occurs as the annulus is stretched further from the papillary muscles. Commercially available tricuspid rings vary in their planar geometry with some being essentially flat, and others having elevation profiles designed to restore normal tricuspid annular height[10] (**Fig. 4**).

Although pulmonary hypertension is certainly an important cause of tricuspid regurgitation, not all patients with pulmonary hypertension exhibit TR. For patients with a systolic pulmonary arterial pressure of 50 to 69 moderate or severe TR is seen in only 35%, and in patients with a PASP of greater than 70 mm Hg moderate or severe TR is seen in 54% demonstrating that there are multiple determinants of TR severity in pulmonary hypertension.[8] Although conceptually it makes sense that in the setting of pulmonary hypertension the increased pressure gradient across the tricuspid valve would be the mechanism for incompetence, a large fraction of patients with pulmonary hypertension have only minimal TR which argues that potentially the mechanism is more related to right ventricular remodeling, annular dilatation, and TV tethering. Although conceptually mitral regurgitation is more closely associated with left ventricular dysfunction approximately 12% of patients with an LV ejection fraction less than 35% will have severe TR, and 30% of patients with severe MR have severe TR. Despite its association with MR, severe TR is an independent predictor of death in patients with LVEF less than 35, with a 1.5 times higher risk of mortality.[5] In these patients with low LVEF, the 1-year survival for those with none to mild TR is 73.4%, 65.9% for those with moderate TR, and 58.7% for those with severe TR.[5]

Renal dysfunction is commonly seen in heart failure patients, occurring to some degree in 50% to 63% of patients,[11,12] and is an important prognostic factor with a 1-year mortality of up to 51% compared to 24% in patients without renal

Fig. 3. Asymmetric annular dilation.[10]

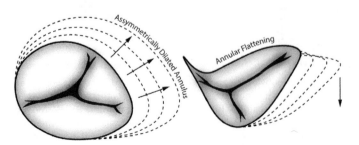

Assymmetrically Dilated Annulus

Annular Flattening

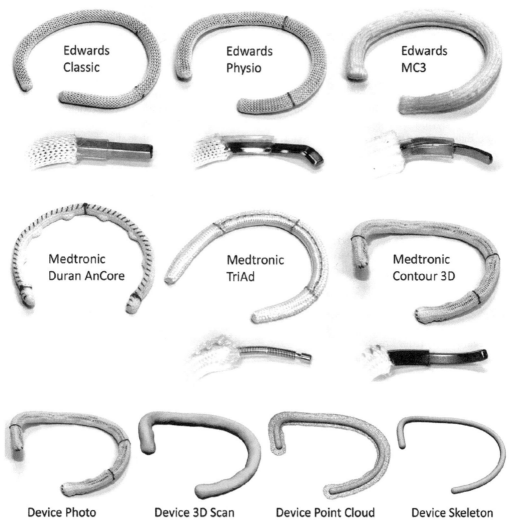

Fig. 4. Some common commercially available rings, cross-section to show device components. 3D scanning can be used to determine ring geometry. From left to right: Edwards Lifesciences (Irvine, CA): Carpentier-Edwards Classic Ring model 4500 (Classic), Carpentier-Edwards Physio Tricuspid Ring model 6200 (Physio), and Edwards MC3 Tricuspid Ring model 4900 (MC3). Medtronic (Minneapolis, MN): Medtronic Duran AnCore Band model 620B (Duran), TriAd Adams Band model 900SFC (TriAd), and Contour 3D Ring model 690R (Contour).[10].

dysfunction.[12] Although typically attributed primarily to low cardiac output or intravascular volume depletion from diuretic therapy, RV dysfunction, tricuspid regurgitation, and the resulting increased renal venous pressure are often overlooked. Elevated CVP alone in a multitude of clinical disorders has been shown to be an independent associate of renal dysfunction.[13] In heart failure patients whose hemodynamics are studied there is an incremental risk of developing worsening renal dysfunction with increasing baseline central venous pressure, 75% of patients with baseline CVP greater than 24 mm Hg developed worsening renal dysfunction during their hospital stay. Similarly, baseline

CVP is significantly higher in patients who develop worsening renal function (18 ± 7 than 12 ± 6)[11]. Interestingly, in this report, the baseline cardiac index was significantly higher in the patients who developed worsening renal failure during their hospitalization and was not found to be a predictor of the development of worsening renal failure. These findings translate to patients with tricuspid regurgitation as expected. Patients with at least moderate TR had lower eGFR, higher BUN, and higher BUN/creatinine ratio than heart failure patients with mild or less TR. And more severe TR was an independent predictor of lower eGFR, higher BUN, and higher BUN/creatinine ratio.[11]

Liver function is also negatively impacted by high venous pressures resulting from heart failure and tricuspid regurgitation. Although typically there is no associated elevation in transaminases as seen in an acute myocardial infarction, hepatopathy secondary to acute decompensated heart failure has a more cholestatic profile. Pulmonary hypertension and degree of LV dysfunction are associated with elevated bilirubin, and severity of TR is also independently associated with elevated alkaline phosphatase, GGT, and bilirubin.[14]

GUIDELINES FOR TRICUSPID SURGERY

Recently released guidelines recommend tricuspid surgery for patients undergoing left-sided valve surgery who have severe TR defined by a central jet $\geq$ 50% RA, vena contracta width $\geq$ 0.7 cm, ERO (effective regurgitant orifice area) ≥ 0.40 cm^2, regurgitant volume $\geq$ 45 mL, dense continuous wave signal with a triangular shape, and hepatic vein systolic flow reversal. Further recommendations for tricuspid valve surgery exist for patients with progressive but not severe TR undergoing left-sided valve surgery who have a dilated tricuspid annulus greater than 4.0 cm in diastole and prior right-sided HF signs tricuspid (level of evidence 2a). For patients with signs and symptoms of right-sided heart failure and severe primary TR or secondary TR that is not responsive to medical therapy, and in the absence of pulmonary hypertension isolated tricuspid valve surgery can be beneficial (level of evidence 2a).[15]

TECHNIQUE

Repair of the tricuspid valve can be approached either via median sternotomy, right thoracotomy or minithoracotomy, or robotically via the right chest. Cardiopulmonary bypass is used, along with bicaval cannulation of the superior and inferior vena cava, and caval snares to isolate the right atrium and to produce as much as possible a bloodless surgical field. The heart can be arrested, or the procedure can be conducted with the heart beating so long as there is no defect in the atrial septum such that air could be entrained into the left side of the heart and ejected through the aortic valve. Exposure of the valve is obtained by opening the right atrium, typically parallel to the atrioventricular groove or toward the tip of the right atrial appendage. If a concomitant mitral procedure is being performed, this is completed first either through the interatrial septum or through a separate incision in the left atrium. The tricuspid commissures are identified. If they are poorly defined or if there are multiple scallops, the ventricular attachments can be of assistance. The valve is tested by injecting saline across the valve to fill the right ventricle and visualize the areas of leak. An appropriately sized band or ring is selected. Traditionally, the teaching is to size the band based on the measurement of the base of the septal leaflet because the septal annulus does not dilate. The size of the ring is also based on the surface area of the leaflet tissue. For functional regurgitation, the size of the ring is usually between 26 and 30 mm. Commercially made band and ring sizers have reference grooves to align with the anteroseptal and posteroseptal commissures to aid in selecting an appropriate size prosthesis. Many different suture techniques can be used but the most common technique is interrupted simple annular sutures using a braided suture. In the case of an incomplete band, the sutures are taken from the anteroseptal commissure around the anterior and posterior annulus, to approximately halfway across the septal leaflet annulus, colloquially from 8 o'clock to 6 o'clock, to avoid the conduction tissue. An appropriately placed band should avoid the area occupied by the AV node and bundle of His, which although not visible to the surgeon, is located on the floor of the right atrium one-third the distance from the coronary sinus to the anteroseptal commissure and the bundle of His follows along the annulus penetrating into the membranous septum. By taking wider stitches on the posterior annulus, you can create symmetric compression to reapproximate normal valve anatomy. After all stitches are taken through the annulus, the band is placed on the annulus and sutures tied. The valve is tested again to ensure competence, and at this point, all leaflets should coapt and there should be a minimal leak if the annulus has been compressed appropriately (Videos 1 and 2).

RESULTS

The introduction of tricuspid rings in the late 1960s improved the management of tricuspid regurgitation significantly. Carpentier reported mortalities of 9.5% and 14% for 150 patients who underwent double valve (mitral and tricuspid) and triple valve (mitral, aortic, and tricuspid) procedures using a tricuspid ring. This is in comparison to the 30% to 48% mortality for patients requiring these procedures using leaflet repair techniques or prosthetic valves.[1]

Although tools for quantifying tricuspid regurgitation were limited in this era and follow-up largely relied on cardiac auscultation and reported symptoms, early studies in the 1970s attempted to determine the optimal management strategy for patients with secondary TR. The De Vega annuloplasty was effective at relieving symptoms from significant TR at up to 14 years in patients with corrected left-sided valvular lesions.[16] In 1985, the first prospective randomized trial of patients with functional TR undergoing repair enrolled 159 patients who were randomized to a De Vega suture annuloplasty or a flexible open ring annuloplasty. At an average of 5 years follow-up in the patients with no residual left-sided valvular dysfunction (80% of the follow-up cohort) 34% of the patients who had received a De Vega annuloplasty had significant TR compared to 10% that had a ring annuloplasty.[17] Suture bicuspidization is technically less challenging, which allows for a shorter bypass and cross-clamp times, and involves typically a single stitch spanning the posterior leaflet which when tied down reduces the orifice area and obliterates the posterior leaflet.[18] Suture bicuspidization has comparable 30 day mortality and echocardiographic results than annuloplasty rings; however, when followed long term, although the survival is equivalent, patients who receive suture bicuspidization have significantly lower freedom from TR recurrence at 1 (91.4% vs 98%), 5 (76.7% vs 86.2%), and 8 years (69.7% vs 73.5%).[19] Although the De Vega suture annuloplasty and suture bicuspidization are still performed in select cases, contemporary repair of functional tricuspid regurgitation is largely comprised of the use of annuloplasty bands.

Contemporary data after echocardiography became widely available and show us that at an average of 5.7 years after surgery patients who receive a ring annuloplasty can have up to an 82% rate of freedom from recurrent TR compared to only 39% who received suture annuloplasty alone.[20] The prevalence of early recurrent moderate or greater TR after surgery is as high as 14% to 23% with severe TR present in up to 10%.[21,22] This early recurrence is similar between rigid rings, flexible bands, and suture annuloplasties up to 6-months post-op. However, after 6 months, the severity of regurgitation remains stable after rigid ring implantation, rises slowly after flexible band implantation, and increases significantly more rapidly after suture annuloplasty. The primary risk factor for early (less than 6 months) recurrence of TR is a high grade of preoperative TR[21,22] and a lower grade of preoperative MR.[18] After

6 months, major risk factors include left ventricular dysfunction, pulmonary hypertension, and the presence of a permanent pacemaker.[21,22] Recurrence rates are reported to be 5% to 8% for severe TR and 17% to 26% for moderate TR at 1 to 3 years[22] and at 6 years 31% of patients have at least moderate TR.[18] In patients with a preoperative permanent pacemaker, the incidence of 3+ or 4+ TR is approximately 16% at 1 month, and 42% at 5 years, than 15% and 23% in those with pacemaker leads traversing the valve. Interestingly, right ventricular systolic pressure, preop functional class, and concomitant surgeries were not risk factors for the development of recurrent TR.[21] Tricuspid valve operations remain a moderately high risk with 30-day mortality around 6% to 9%,[18] 5-year survival 65%, and 8-year survival 50%. Reoperation for recurrent TR has a high mortality as one would expect, up to 35% 30-day mortality, and the risk of reoperation is 4.2% per year for the first 3 years.[21,23]

In patients undergoing the repair of a degenerative mitral valve the question of how to treat tricuspid regurgitation is a subject of debate. Practices vary widely with reported rates of concomitant tricuspid repair ranging from 10% to 63%.[24–26] Proponents of a conservative approach argue that after correcting left-sided lesions, the RV loading conditions improve and subsequently TR will improve,[27] and that mortality is unaffected with this approach.[27] This, however, is contradictory to the data that suggest that in isolation TR decreases survival.[4] Most data on the subject come from observational studies, and the decision to repair the tricuspid valve is highly variable. Typically, the patients have similar baseline characteristics, demographics, and echocardiographic parameters between those that undergo TV repair and those that don't;[28,29] however, some series show a higher incidence of biventricular dysfunction in the group with more severe TR that ultimately undergoes repair,[25] which is congruent with the physiologic explanation of right ventricular remodeling altering the tricuspid annulus which in turn causes insufficiency. Regardless of the functional status of the ventricles, the perioperative mortality is similar if the tricuspid is repaired or if the valve is left alone.[25,28,29] Tricuspid annuloplasty in the setting of left-sided valve surgery has comparable results to isolated annuloplasty with only 5% moderate TR and 2% severe TR at an average of 14-months follow-up.[30] Although there are no randomized trials to address the question, propensity-matched groups in observational trials show an improved 5-year survival in those patients who had a tricuspid repair, 74.5% compared to 45% in those whose TR was untreated.[28] In patients who undergo tricuspid annuloplasty, pulmonary artery pressures improve and right atrial size decreases. Although RV function may initially worsen, at follow-up tricuspid annuloplasty has been shown to be an independent positive predictor of late RV recovery.[25] Additionally, there is a benefit to functional status at 5 years as well with 60% of tricuspid repair patients being alive and NYHA I or II at year compared to 39.8% for those who did not have a tricuspid repair.[28]

What to do in the case of a dilated annulus but less than severe TR poses an additional subject of debate. More aggressive surgeons argue that tricuspid annular dilation is a permanent change and does not reverse after correcting left-sided valve disease, and even a competent valve in the setting of a dilated annulus will degenerate over time and become regurgitant.[29] The converse argument made is that many of the patients with degenerative disease have myxomatous leaflets which are able to maintain competence in a dilated annulus.[31] In a report from a single high-volume center where concomitant tricuspid annuloplasty was completed when the tricuspid annulus was greater than 40 mm, the patients who had mild preoperative TR with a large annulus treated with an annuloplasty ring had a significantly higher freedom from moderate TR at 7 years than those who started with mild TR and who did not receive an annuloplasty ring (97% vs 83%).[25] In contrast when a different high-volume center managed moderate or less TR conservatively during mitral valve surgery and reported their postoperative outcomes stratified based on a preoperative tricuspid annular measurements, they found no association between preoperative a tricuspid annulus greater than 40 mm and degree of postoperative TR.[31] Currently, a randomized study evaluating tricuspid repair versus conservative management during concomitant mitral repair for degenerative disease is ongoing. This trial will randomize patients with either moderate TR or less than moderate TR with an annulus greater than 40 mm, and we are currently awaiting the 2-year clinical and echocardiographic results.

Progression of functional TR after the mitral repair is not related to the recurrence or progression of mitral regurgitation and progression to moderate or severe TR is seen in up to 45% of patients after mitral repair.[20,28] For patients with mild TR who undergo mitral surgery, 37% progress to moderate or worse TR at an average of 8 years follow-up.[32] Atrial fibrillation and a large left atrium are risk factors for TR recurrence after mitral valve surgery, as is more than mild preoperative TR.[32]

TRICUSPID REPLACEMENT

Historically during the advent of surgical therapy for tricuspid valve disease, the treatment of mild TR, as determined by preoperative catheterization or intraoperative digital examination, was conservative management, moderate TR was treated with an annuloplasty, and severe TR was treated with tricuspid replacement.[16,33] In the current era with more techniques and implants available for annuloplasty, tricuspid valve replacement is relatively uncommon. Society of Thoracic Surgeons indicates that 89% of tricuspid interventions are repaired, and 86% are performed concomitantly with another major procedure.[34] However, in the case of isolated tricuspid pathology necessitating surgery replacements are more common. From 2004 to 2013, the largest publicly available database in the United States reported that of patients who required an isolated tricuspid intervention, 41% had their valve repaired than 59% were replaced (61% bioprosthetic, and 39% mechanical). Mortality is relatively high for these operations, and significantly greater for patients who required replacement: 5.9% for tricuspid repair, 9.1% for bioprosthetic valves, and 13.6% for mechanical valves.[35]

SUMMARY

The tricuspid valve is an often forgotten but relevant cause of significant morbidity and mortality. Serious consideration should be given to addressing the valve in patients undergoing left-sided valve surgery who have functional TR, or an enlarged annulus. Tricuspid repair with a ring annuloplasty has shown improved long-term survival and freedom from recurrent TR at as long as 15 years of follow-up compared to suture annuloplasty or other repairs whereby a prosthetic ring is not used.

CLINICS CARE POINTS

- 1.6 million Americans have moderate to severe TR; however, tricuspid valve procedures are relatively uncommon representing only 3% of cardiac surgeries performed today.

- Annular dilation is not symmetric. The posterior leaflet is the most severely affected and can increase up to 80% of its annular length. The anterior leaflet can see a 40% increase in length, and the septal leaflet, which is largely unaffected due to its attachment to the interventricular septum, sees only a 10% increase.

- How to manage a dilated tricuspid annulus is patients undergoing left sided valve surgery remains a topic of great debate. Some studies show improved survival at 5 years (74.5% vs 45%), and improved functional status (60% NYHA I or II vs 39.8%) for those who undergo tricuspid repair at the time of left sided valve surgery.

DISCLOSURE

Dr A.A. Jonsson - NONE. Dr M.E. Halkos – Medtronic – serve on their Advisory Board.

SUPPLEMENTARY DATA

Supplementary data related to this article can be found online at https://doi.org/10.1016/j.iccl.2021.09.007.

REFERENCES

1. Carpentier A, Deloche A, Hanania G, et al. Surgical management of acquired tricuspid valve disease. J Thorac Cardiovasc Surg 1974;67(1):53–65.
2. Stuge O, Liddicoat J. Emerging opportunities for cardiac surgeons within structural heart disease. J Thorac Cardiovasc Surg 2006;132(6):1258–61.
3. D'Agostino RS, Jacobs JP, Badhwar V, et al. The Society of Thoracic Surgeons Adult Cardiac Surgery Database: 2016 Update on Outcomes and Quality. Ann Thorac Surg 2016;101(1):24–32.
4. Nath J, Foster E, Heidenreich PA. Impact of tricuspid regurgitation on long-term survival. J Am Coll Cardiol 2004;43(3):405–9.
5. Koelling TM, Aaronson KD, Cody RJ, et al. Prognostic significance of mitral regurgitation and tricuspid regurgitation in patients with left ventricular systolic dysfunction. Am Heart J 2002;144(3):524–9.
6. Agricola E, Marini C, Stella S, et al. Effects of functional tricuspid regurgitation on renal function and long-term prognosis in patients with heart failure. J Cardiovasc Med (Hagerstown) 2017;18(2):60–8.
7. Kawada N, Naganuma H, Muramatsu K, et al. Redefinition of tricuspid valve structures for successful ring annuloplasty. J Thorac Cardiovasc Surg 2018;155(4):1511–9.e1.
8. Mutlak D, Aronson D, Lessick J, et al. Functional tricuspid regurgitation in patients with pulmonary hypertension: is pulmonary artery pressure the only determinant of regurgitation severity? Chest 2009;135(1):115–21.
9. Ton-Nu TT, Levine RA, Handschumacher MD, et al. Geometric determinants of functional tricuspid regurgitation: insights from 3-dimensional echocardiography. Circulation 2006;114(2):143–9.
10. Mathur M, Malinowski M, Timek TA, et al. Tricuspid Annuloplasty Rings: A Quantitative Comparison of Size, Nonplanar Shape, and Stiffness. Ann Thorac Surg 2020;110(5):1605–14.
11. Maeder MT, Holst DP, Kaye DM. Tricuspid regurgitation contributes to renal dysfunction in patients with heart failure. J Card Fail 2008;14(10):824–30.
12. Smith GL, Lichtman JH, Bracken MB, et al. Renal impairment and outcomes in heart failure: systematic review and meta-analysis. J Am Coll Cardiol 2006;47(10):1987–96.
13. Damman K, van Deursen VM, Navis G, et al. Increased central venous pressure is associated with impaired renal function and mortality in a broad spectrum of patients with cardiovascular disease. J Am Coll Cardiol 2009;53(7):582–8.
14. Lau GT, Tan HC, Kritharides L. Type of liver dysfunction in heart failure and its relation to the severity of tricuspid regurgitation. Am J Cardiol 2002;90(12):1405–9.
15. Otto CM, Nishimura RA, Bonow RO, et al. 2020 ACC/AHA Guideline for the Management of Patients With Valvular Heart Disease: Executive Summary: A Report of the American College of Cardiology/American Heart Association Joint Committee on Clinical Practice Guidelines. Circulation 2021;143(5):e35–71.
16. Chidambaram M, Abdulali SA, Baliga BG, et al. Long-term results of DeVega tricuspid annuloplasty. Ann Thorac Surg 1987;43(2):185–8.
17. Rivera R, Duran E, Ajuria M. Carpentier's flexible ring versus De Vega's annuloplasty. A prospective randomized study. J Thorac Cardiovasc Surg 1985;89(2):196–203.
18. Ghanta RK, Chen R, Narayanasamy N, et al. Suture bicuspidization of the tricuspid valve versus ring annuloplasty for repair of functional tricuspid regurgitation: midterm results of 237 consecutive patients. J Thorac Cardiovasc Surg 2007;133(1):117–26.
19. Hirji S, Yazdchi F, Kiehm S, et al. Outcomes After Tricuspid Valve Repair With Ring Versus Suture Bicuspidization Annuloplasty. Ann Thorac Surg 2020;110(3):821–8.
20. Tang GH, David TE, Singh SK, et al. Tricuspid valve repair with an annuloplasty ring results in improved long-term outcomes. Circulation 2006 Jul 4;114(1 Suppl):I577–81.
21. McCarthy PM, Bhudia SK, Rajeswaran J, et al. Tricuspid valve repair: durability and risk factors for failure. J Thorac Cardiovasc Surg 2004;127(3):674–85.

22. Fukuda S, Gillinov AM, McCarthy PM, et al. Determinants of recurrent or residual functional tricuspid regurgitation after tricuspid annuloplasty. Circulation 2006;114(1 Suppl):I582–7.

23. Bernal JM, Morales D, Revuelta C, et al. Reoperations after tricuspid valve repair. J Thorac Cardiovasc Surg 2005;130(2):498–503.

24. Gillinov AM, Mihaljevic T, Blackstone EH, et al. Should patients with severe degenerative mitral regurgitation delay surgery until symptoms develop? Ann Thorac Surg 2010;90(2):481–8.

25. Chikwe J, Itagaki S, Anyanwu A, et al. Impact of Concomitant Tricuspid Annuloplasty on Tricuspid Regurgitation, Right Ventricular Function, and Pulmonary Artery Hypertension After Repair of Mitral Valve Prolapse. J Am Coll Cardiol 2015;65(18): 1931–8.

26. Castillo JG, Anyanwu AC, Fuster V, et al. A near 100% repair rate for mitral valve prolapse is achievable in a reference center: implications for future guidelines. J Thorac Cardiovasc Surg 2012;144(2):308–12.

27. Yilmaz O, Suri RM, Dearani JA, et al. Functional tricuspid regurgitation at the time of mitral valve repair for degenerative leaflet prolapse: the case for a selective approach. J Thorac Cardiovasc Surg 2011;142(3):608–13.

28. Calafiore AM, Gallina S, Iacò AL, et al. Mitral valve surgery for functional mitral regurgitation: should moderate-or-more tricuspid regurgitation be treated? a propensity score analysis. Ann Thorac Surg 2009;87(3):698–703.

29. Dreyfus GD, Corbi PJ, Chan KM, et al. Secondary tricuspid regurgitation or dilatation: which should be the criteria for surgical repair? Ann Thorac Surg 2005;79(1):127–32.

30. Brescia AA, Ward ST, Watt TMF, et al. Outcomes of Guideline-Directed Concomitant Annuloplasty for Functional Tricuspid Regurgitation. Ann Thorac Surg 2020;109(4):1227–32.

31. David TE, David CM, Manlhiot C. Tricuspid annulus diameter does not predict the development of tricuspid regurgitation after mitral valve repair for mitral regurgitation due to degenerative diseases. J Thorac Cardiovasc Surg 2018;155(6):2429–36.

32. Matsuyama K, Matsumoto M, Sugita T, et al. Predictors of residual tricuspid regurgitation after mitral valve surgery. Ann Thorac Surg 2003;75(6):1826–8.

33. Breyer RH, McClenathan JH, Michaelis LL, et al. Tricuspid regurgitation. A comparison of nonoperative management, tricuspid annuloplasty, and tricuspid valve replacement. J Thorac Cardiovasc Surg 1976;72(6):867–74.

34. Kilic A, Saha-Chaudhuri P, Rankin JS, et al. Trends and outcomes of tricuspid valve surgery in North America: an analysis of more than 50,000 patients from the Society of Thoracic Surgeons database. Ann Thorac Surg 2013;96(5):1546–52.

35. Zack CJ, Fender EA, Chandrashekar P, et al. National Trends and Outcomes in Isolated Tricuspid Valve Surgery. J Am Coll Cardiol 2017;70(24): 2953–60.

Transcatheter Leaflet Strategies for Tricuspid Regurgitation TriClip and CLASP

Johanna Vogelhuber, MD, Marcel Weber, MD,
Georg Nickenig, MD*

KEYWORDS

- Tricuspid regurgitation • Right heart failure • Tricuspid annulus • Tricuspid valve • TTVr
- Transcatheter tricuspid valve repair • Leaflet approximation devices • TEER

KEY POINTS

- Significant TR is associated with poor clinical outcome and treatment of significant TR (with optimal heart failure therapy as well as additional surgical/interventional treatment) can improve clinical symptoms.
- Thus far, the most common catheter-based treatment options are leaflet approximation devices for transcatheter edge-to-edge repair (TEER), such as TriClip (Abbott, Santa Clara, CA, USA) and the PASCAL Implant System (Edwards Lifesciences, Irvine, CA, USA).
- Both, TriClip and PASCAL Implant System proved to be feasible, safe, and efficient in reducing TR and improving clinical and echocardiographic outcome parameters with low peri-interventional complication rates and serve as a viable treatment option for patients at high surgical risk.

Tricuspid regurgitation (TR) is a common finding and can frequently be observed during routine echocardiography—as an incidental finding or as a consequence of leading left-sided heart diseases (as secondary TR).[1] The population-based Framingham Heart Study showed a prevalence of mild TR in overall greater than 80% of the population—particularly affecting people at older age and of female gender.[2] Consequently and with regard to the elderly (>70 years), a significant TR (≥moderate) was present in 1%,5% of male and 5%, 6% of female patients, respectively.[2] Moreover, prevalence of ≥moderate TR in patients with chronic heart failure and reduced left ventricular ejection fraction is even higher with approximately 26%.[2–4] The importance of TR for prognosis has long been underrated and treatment has subsequently been neglected in accordance with initial recommendations to handle TR conservatively with optimal heart failure therapy.[5–7] As a consequence, progressive TR left untreated can entail tricuspid annular dilation, right ventricular (RV) dilation and right heart failure with RV overload which itself worsens TR in a negative loop. Especially significant secondary TR (STR) comprises greater than 80% of TR cases[8,9]) can long remain silent, compensated, and asymptomatic—but might still be progressing—despite the treatment of potentially accompanied left-sided valvular diseases, thus, complicating the treatment and decision-making process. Moreover, STR—particularly refractory STR—stands as a marker for progressed heart failure with unfavorable outcome, high morbidity, and mortality.[4,5,10–12] In particular, preinterventional STR in patients after transcatheter mitral valve repair only improved postinterventional in roughly one-third and persisting or even progressing STR was simultaneously associated with worse

Heart Centre, Department of Cardiology, University Hospital Bonn, Sigmund-Freud-Str. 25, 53127 Bonn, Germany
* Corresponding author. Heart Centre, Department of Cardiology, University Hospital Bonn, Sigmund-Freud-Street, 25, Bonn 53127, Germany.
E-mail address: georg.nickenig@ukbonn.de

Intervent Cardiol Clin 11 (2022) 51–66
https://doi.org/10.1016/j.iccl.2021.09.005
2211-7458/22/© 2021 Elsevier Inc. All rights reserved.

outcome.[13,14] Given the fact that the demographic change results in a near doubling of the population greater than 65 years of age until 2050,[5,15] management of significant TR will pose a growing challenge for general practitioners and cardiologists. In addition, conventional (surgical) TV reconstruction or replacement is associated with a comparatively high perioperative mortality with reports showing an in-hospital mortality of up to 10%.[8,16] Moreover, the comparatively late referral to the specific treatment of those often older and multimorbid patients at high surgical risk has increased the need for less invasive treatment options, thus, the development of minimally invasive and catheter-based treatment strategies has, therefore, come to the fore to offer the growing patient collective at high surgical risk—mainly due to advanced age and multiple comorbidities—effective and personalized therapy options.

EXCURSUS: ANATOMY OF SECONDARY TRICUSPID REGURGITATION

TR is mainly secondary (>80%) and mostly associated with and the consequence of a leading left-sided heart pathology with subsequent congestive heart failure.[1] Only 8% to 10% of TR are thought to be primary (organic).

The tricuspid valve is the most complex valve and its anatomy is more heterogenous than generally anticipated: contrary to what its name might suggest, the tricuspid valve consists only in 57% of 3 leaflets.[17,18] In 43% one can find at least 4 leaflets with one additional leaflet mostly between the septal and posterior leaflet.[17,18] As typically for atrioventricular valves, the tricuspid valve has a three-dimensional, saddle-shaped, elliptical geometry with a pliant, noncircular and comparatively large annulus. Since the septal portion is rather fibrous and the anterior and posterior portion rather muscular, annular dilation in the context of secondary TR usually occurs along the anteroseptal to posteroseptal commissure.[17] In cases of progressed secondary TR with pronounced annular dilation, leaflet tethering and tenting of especially the septal leaflet can be observed. Various notable structures are in close proximity surrounding the tricuspid valve, one of which is most importantly the right coronary artery (RCA) passing along the tricuspid annulus from anterior to posterior with its ostium anteroseptal.[17] The Koch Triangle (with AV node and His Bundle) and the coronary sinus are both posteroseptal of the tricuspid annulus[17]; hence, tricuspid valve interventions pose a great challenge as variable valve morphology and surrounding structures complicate each procedure.

Of note, anatomic variations such as scallops, folds, or incisions within the leaflets further pose notable challenges concerning the grasping process during transcatheter edge-to-edge repair (TEER) and need to be assessed closely during preinterventional evaluation—especially with transoesophageal echocardiography—and those anatomic circumstances need to be taken into account regarding individual device selection.

Further insight into the specific anatomy and pathophysiology of secondary TR are included in Section 1 of this issue, Fig. 1 provides an illustration of the main pathophysiology of secondary TR.

More information regarding preinterventional imaging (TTE, TOE, CT, MRI) crucial for the optimal preparation of transcatheter tricuspid valve repair (TTVr) as well as information concerning TR grading can be found in Sections 2 and 3 of this issue.

THERAPEUTIC TREATMENT OPTIONS

For decision-making in terms of the optimal treatment regimen of significant symptomatic TR, the present etiology and differentiation between primary, secondary, and isolated TR, respectively, must be taken into account.

As the significance of transcatheter treatment options for patients with primary TR is up to now rather negligible,[19–21] the focus will be on treatment strategies for secondary TR.

Optimal medical heart failure therapy is the cornerstone of any treatment concept for patients with secondary TR and, mostly, affects positively course and development of functional TR.[22] Early references from the 1960 primarily suggested a rather conservative treatment strategy leading to an overall negligence of TR and to its nickname the forgotten valve.[5,6] Progressive and significant functional TR—even after effective left-heart valve therapy—is a marker for progressing chronic heart failure and is associated with considerably higher morbidity and mortality, thus, with worse outcome.

Up to now, for patients with symptomatic and progressive TR (≥severe) despite optimal medical heart failure therapy, ESC Guidelines state a Class I-recommendation (Level of evidence B) for surgical treatment if a simultaneous left-sided heart surgery is indicated (eg, AS, MR and/or CABG).[19,21] In this context, the extent of tricuspid annulus dilation is of particular interest regarding procedural planning, meaning a

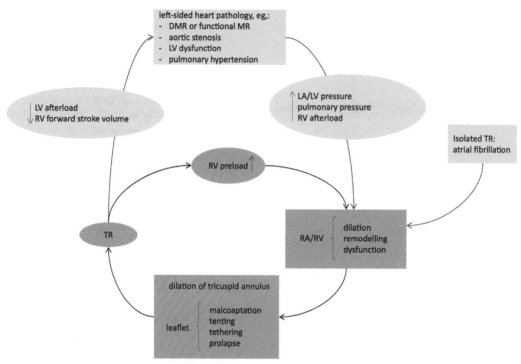

Fig. 1. Pathomechanisms of functional TR. DMR, degenerative mitral regurgitation; LA, left atrium; LV, left ventricle; MR, mitral regurgitation; RA, right atrium; RV, right ventricle; TR, tricuspid regurgitation.

more pronounced annular dilation (≥40 mm or >21 mm/m²)—even with mild or moderate TR—should more liberally be considered for surgical treatment (Class IIa-recommendation, Level of evidence B).[21] Additionally, the degree of RV dilation and recent right heart failure have to be taken into account as well while careful weighing of therapeutic options to prevent further progression of TR and worse outcome. Due to the comparatively high perioperative risk with a significantly increased mortality and morbidity in patients with significant TR and previous heart surgery, a renewed surgical intervention should be evaluated critically—correspondingly ESC Guidelines only state a Class IIa-recommendation (Level of evidence B) for the surgical intervention of symptomatic STR in patients with a history of previous heart surgery.[21] Furthermore, with surgical treatment of isolated TR (≥severe) showing the highest perioperative mortality of all heart-valve surgeries,[23] there has been a change of course regarding the overall treatment recommendations for functional TR during the past decade: Firstly, an earlier treatment is recommended to prevent excess mortality and morbidity due to severe STR; secondly, the development of

minimal-invasive, catheter-based therapies has come to focus to offer the growing population at high surgical risk with increased morbidity and contraindications for surgical intervention alternative treatment options with a justifiable benefit-risk-ratio. This led to the subsequent inclusion of transcatheter treatment options for symptomatic, severe STR in the newly updated ESC/EACTS Guidelines for management of valvular heart disease (Class IIb-recommendation, Level of evidence C).[21] As a sidenote, there have been noteworthy improvements in surgical techniques as well allowing for minimally invasive surgery or surgery on beating heart to improve complication rate and perioperative risk.

Nonetheless, there is a great interest in minimal-invasive and catheter-based treatment strategies for the growing cohort of patients with significant functional TR at high-surgical risk with contraindications for surgical intervention. Presently, there are numerous catheter-based therapies available—some of them have already been proven to be safe, effective, and beneficial, others are still under evaluation and only accessible for compassionate use or within clinical trials. Some of the said interventional procedures were initially developed and established for the treatment of mitral valve regurgitation and have later been adapted for the tricuspid valve. Generally, these procedures are classified in terms of their approach and effect mechanism:

- edge-to-edge-repair (leaflet coaptation devices)
- direct ring-annuloplasty (repair)
- transcatheter valve replacement

REQUIREMENTS FOR TRANSCATHETER EDGE-TO-EDGE REPAIR

Patients with STR—significant, symptomatic, and/or progressive despite guideline-directed optimal heart failure therapy and/or adequate prior treatment of left-sided heart diseases (eg, coronary artery disease [CAD], mitral regurgitation [MR], aortic stenosis [AS])—might benefit from additional interventional care of STR. In preparation for and to further evaluate an individually suitable interventional approach, a detailed examination including functional capacity (6-min-walking-test [6MWT], body plethysmography/diffusion capacity), clinical assessment, evaluation of potential extracardial artery diseases and left-/right-heart catheterization is obligatory,—particularly to estimate procedural success, risk, and outcome, respectively. The cornerstone of any preprocedural assessment, however, is transthoracic and above all, transoesophageal echocardiography (TTE, TOE; 2D and 3D). TOE allows for a further and more detailed display of the tricuspid valve, its subvalvular apparatus, and leaflets and is crucial for a proper characterization of 1) present pathologies (eg, number of leaflets, scallops/folds/incisures, leaflet tenting/tethering/prolapse, flail leaflet), 2) the size and localization of the precise coaptation defect and its configuration, and 3) for procedural planning. Multiplane and 3D TOE contribute additional valuable insight (Figs. 2 and 3). Complementary 3D images with added color Doppler enable planimetric measuring of VC and EROA (see Fig. 3).[24] Due to the complex anatomy of the tricuspid valve, the informative value, and validity of TOE is variable and particularly dependent on the examiner's expertise and experience, thus, TOE in the scope of procedure evaluation and planning mainly occurs in a specialized core laboratory. Limitations of echocardiography (2D/3D TOE/TTE) consist in the insufficient imaging planes of the contiguous cardiovascular anatomy (ie, superior vena cava, inferior vena

cava), its limited display of RV and RA anatomy, and low three-dimensional resolution.

High-resolution ECG-triggered cardiac CT (cCT) functions as an important and central diagnostic tool regarding the selection of the individually suitable treatment strategy and preprocedural planning and simulation. The main strength certainly is its high three-dimensional resolution for optimal assessment of RA and RV volume and anatomy, of the valvular apparatus, surrounding structures (eg, right ventricular outflow tract [ROVT], RCA, trabecula), and the afferent/efferent vessels (access routes), as well as for the calculation of RV forward stroke volume.[24–26] Potential pacemaker- or ICD-leads may cause relevant artifacts limiting the informative value of cCT significantly. Moreover, tachycardia such as atrial fibrillation may cause a significant quality loss, too, for which even an ECG-triggered scheme cannot compensate.[24–26]

More detailed information regarding preprocedural imaging and TR grading can be found in Sections 2 and 3 of this issue.

Every patient in planning for TR treatment will be presented and discussed in an interdisciplinary heart team; in this context, conventional scoring systems such as EuroSCORE II and STS Score are still applied in terms of the assessment of periprocedural risk. It needs to be mentioned that these scoring systems—originally designed for left-sided heart diseases—are sometimes misleading as they do not include parameters for right heart function and failure, respectively, and thus, tend to underestimate the periprocedural risk for right heart procedures. Consequently, in this context, they should be used with caution and rated critically.

PROCEDURAL SETTING

Minimally invasive, transcatheter tricuspid valve repair requires a cath lab or hybrid operation room with fluoroscopy and TOE imaging and is performed under general anesthesia, thus, an interventionalist, an imager and, an anesthesiologist with their respective assisting staff (eg, for device preparation and for support during device navigation and handling) ought to be present. However, the presence of a heart surgeon in the facility is not required, nonetheless, prior interdisciplinary heart team decision includes an assessment of a trained heart surgeon. For TEER with either device—TriClip or PASCAL Implant System—a 22 to 24F transfemoral-venous assess route is used with intravenous application of Heparin aiming for

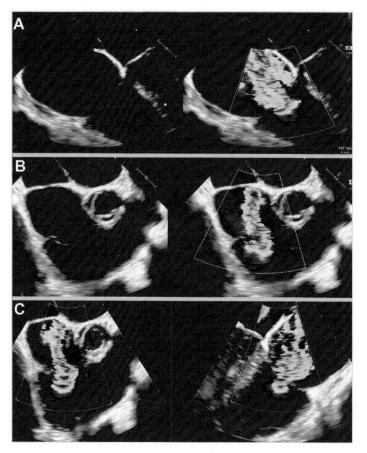

Fig. 2. TOE: TR. (*A*) 4-Chamber view (+/− color Doppler); (*B*) commissural view (inflow/outflow view, +/− color Doppler), (*C*) left: commissural view + color Doppler, right: grasping view (reversed 4-chamber view) + color Doppler.

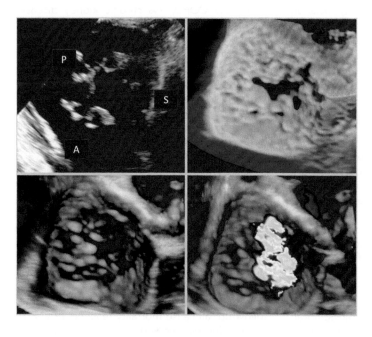

Fig. 3. TOE: Tricuspid valve. Upper left: transgastric view, other: 3-dimensional reconstruction ± color doppler. A, anterior; P, posterior; S, septal.

an ACT (activated clotting time) between 250 to 350 seconds.

TREATMENT STRATEGIES FOR TRANSCATHETER EDGE-TO-EDGE REPAIR

Regarding the choice of individual treatment strategy, 2 approaches have been proposed and validated in several trials and reports[8,26–31]; one of which is attempting *bicuspidalization* of the tricuspid valve in *zipping technique* by placing the first device in far anteroseptal position and the following devices along the anteroseptal commissure inwards (rarely the same strategy can be applied starting from the posteroseptal commissure inwards). The other proposed approach is creating a *triple orifice* whereby the first device is usually placed in the anteroseptal commissure in rather central position and the second in posteroseptal position which subsequently creates a *triple orifice*. With both techniques being regularly applied, *bicuspidalization* in *zipping technique* is used more frequently as in patients with significant functional TR localization of coaptation defect is mainly observed in anteroseptal position due to pronounced right heart and tricuspid annular dilation and volume overload and since—as mentioned above—enlargement of the tricuspid annulus mainly occurs along the anteroseptal to posteroseptal commissure. **Figs. 4** and **5** display an example of the proposed *zipping technique* leading to a bicuspidalization of the tricuspid valve. **Fig. 6** shows an example of a *triple orifice*.

The following paragraphs especially focus on the 2 most common leaflet approximation devices for edge-to-edge tricuspid valve repair (TEER), TriClip (Abbott, Santa Clara, CA, USA), and PASCAL Implant System (Edwards Lifesciences, Irvine, CA, USA).

MitraClip/TriClip (ABBOTT, SANTA CLARA, CA, USA)

Initially, the MitraClip device was established as a promising catheter-based procedure for both degenerative and functional mitral regurgitation for high-risk patients[26,27]; subsequently, this validated technique was adapted for treating secondary TR and up to now, the Mitraclip device and its adaption for the tricuspid valve—Tri-Clip[32]—have been used most frequently in regards to transcatheter TEER for treatment of TR (eg, 80% of patients included in the TriValve Registry,[8,33]).

The device is deployed via transfemoralvenous 22F-delivery system and consists of a steerable guide catheter and a clip delivery system. Especially anteroseptal and posteroseptal coaptation defects can be approached and treated successfully with the redefined *TriClip* which has received a CE mark in 2020. In this context, one or more clips can be implanted—generating either a *bicuspidalization* if clips are positioned along the anteroseptal *or* posteroseptal commissure in *zipping technique* or a *triple orifice* if clips are positioned anteroseptal *and* posteroseptal[26–30]—as mentioned above. The *TriClip* is available in 2 different sizes—NT and XT—the bigger XT-device allows the treatment of bigger and more complex coaptation defects (eg, leaflet prolapse or tenting).[26,27,29,30] **Fig. 7** gives an overview of the main characteristics and features of the TriClip device. Feasibility, safety, and efficacy had already been proven during the first clinical trials documenting a procedural success rate of greater than 95% with a significant TR reduction ($\geq$1 grade) and improved clinical outcome (NYHA Class, 6-MWT, KCCQ).[31,34–38] Mehr and colleagues included 249 patients with symptomatic TR treated with TTVr with MitraClip in the multicenter TriValve Registry between 2015 and 2018.[31] The included patients were in average 77 years of age, female in 51% and at high surgical risk as represented by an EuroSCORE II of 6%,4%. NYHA Class was $\geq$III in 94%, patients were multimorbid with 74% atrial fibrillation, 68% concomitant left-sided valvular diseases, 30% presence of a permanent pacemaker or ICD, 26% reduced left ventricular ejection fraction, 25% COPD, 7% chronic kidney disease, and 30% diabetes mellitus. TR grade was greater than 3 in 45% and greater than 4 in 52%, respectively, and mainly secondary (89%). Technical success rate was 96% with 2 implanted devices per procedure on average—in 86% in anteroseptal position and 21% anteroseptal and posteroseptal, respectively. Procedural success was achieved in 77% (TR reduction to $\leq$2+) and 89% (TR reduction of 1 grade to baseline), respectively. The portion of patients with TR grade $\geq$3 was reduced from 97% at baseline to 23% and 28% at discharge and 1-year follow-up, respectively. Of note, 52% of patients were treated simultaneously for concomitant significant mitral regurgitation in one procedure with edge-to-edge mitral valve repair. There were no periprocedural deaths, although 3 patients died within the initial hospital stay, there was 1 conversion to open-heart surgery and 2 strokes in patients with concomitant TMVR. At 1-year follow-up, all-cause mortality reached 19%. Procedural success showed a significant impact on

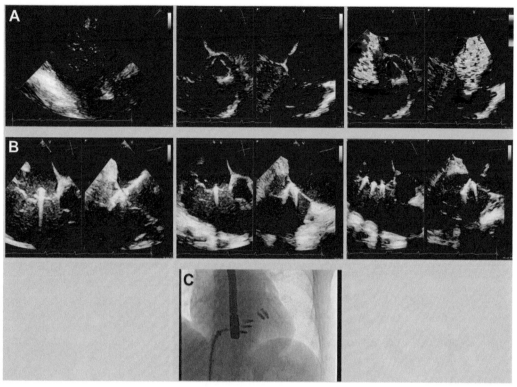

Fig. 4. Edge-to-edge tricuspid valve repair in zipping technique (bicuspidalization). (*A*) Preinterventional imaging: left: transgastrical view; middle/, biplane: commissural view + grasping view; right, biplane: commissural view + grasping view + color Doppler. (*B*) device deployment: left, biplane: commissural view + grasping view with 1 TriClip XT deployed (still attached to the delivery system); left, biplane: commissural view + grasping view with 3 deployed TriClip XT, already detached. (*C*) Periinterventional fluoroscopy: 3 deployed TriClip XT, delivery system, and TOE probe, also: 2 PA Ace Implant Systems in the mitral position.

1-year mortality and the need for rehospitalization. Regarding functional outcome, NYHA Class was improved at least 1 grade in 72% of patients, 69% of patients were NYHA Class I + II (compared with 5% at baseline).

Subsequently, the prospective, multi-center, and single-arm study TRILUMINATE was initiated for further analysis. Typically, the included 85 patients were older (mean age 77,8), more often female (66%), multimorbid (eg, 92% atrial fibrillation, 86% arterial hypertension, 46% renal impairment, 33% previous mitral intervention, 22% diabetes mellitus, 18% previous myocardial infarction) and at high surgical risk as represented by an average EuroScore II of 8%,6%. With an implant success of 100% (=successful deployment), TR was reduced by at least 1 grade at discharge in 91% (76 patients) and in 86% at 30 days follow-up. In this trial, the five-scaled grading scheme by Hahn and colleagues was applied.[24,39] At 6-month follow-up the proportion of patients with severe TR was reduced

to 24% (29% at baseline), while 7% (29% at baseline) and 1% (37% at baseline) showed massive or torrential TR at 6-month follow-up, respectively. Correspondingly, a significant functional improvement (NYHA Class, 6-MWT, KCCQ) at 30 days and 6-month follow-up was observed.[32] In average, 2,2 devices were implanted per procedure, mainly in the anteroseptal commissure (77%, 20% posteroseptal). Regarding the primary safety endpoint, no device embolization, stroke, or myocardial infarction was reported; single leaflet device detachment (SLDA) was observed in 5 patients (7%), and in 6 patients the mean gradient across the tricuspid valve was >5 mm Hg at 6-month follow-up indicating tricuspid stenosis. Regarding safety endpoints, 30 day survival was 100% and all-cause mortality at 6 months came to 5% (n = 4) with 2% (n = 2) cardiovascular deaths. Echocardiographic follow-up after 6 months showed an improvement of RV function (TAPSE, RV fractional area change [RV FAC]) and extend of RA and RV

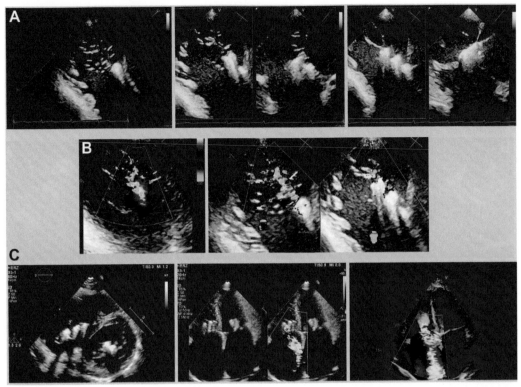

Fig. 5. Edge-to-edge- tricuspid valve repair in zipping technique. (*A*) Transgastrical view (+biplane): left: 1 TriClip XT far anteroseptal; middle: 2 TriClip XT; right: 3 TriClip XT from far anteroseptal to central; highlighted as dashed circle: bicuspidalized tricuspid valve as single orifice. (*B*) Transgastrical view + color Doppler: left: preinterventional; middle: 1 TriClip XT; right: 3 TriClip XT deployed. (*C*) Postinterventional TTE: left: parasternal short axis: 2 TriClip XT, also 2 PACSAL Ace Implant System in mitral position; middle: 4-chamber view ± color Doppler; right: preinterventional 4-chamber view + color Doppler for comparison.

dilation, thus, suggesting the TriClip procedure as a safe and effective treatment option for STR in high-risk patients.[32] The recent publication of the 1-year follow-up showed a persisting TR reduction (TR ≤ moderate in 71% at 1-year follow-up, 8% at Baseline). Moreover, NYHA Class was ≤II in 83% (31% at baseline). Mortality and major adverse events were 7%. Regarding echocardiographic parameters, RV and RA size and function were significantly improved indicating reverse RV remodeling after TTVr.[40]

Similar to the PASCAL Implant System, an evolution of the TriClip device can be expected with the technical option of independent grasping (comparable to the MitraClip Generation 4)—prospectively within the next months to come.

Further trials are ongoing to assess TTVr with the TriClip device—especially compared with optimal medical therapy (OMT); of particular note in this context are the TRILUMINATE Pivotal Trial (NCT03904147) and the TRICuspid Intervention in Heart Failure Trial (NCT04634266).

PASCAL implant system (Edwards Lifesciences, Irvine, CA, USA)

Similar to the TriClip device, the PASCAL Implant was first established for the treatment of mitral regurgitation.[41–43] Otherwise similar in design, the PASCAL Implant is bigger and features separately steerable paddles and an additional central spacer for optimal sealing of the coaptation defect.[31,41,44] The increased span width and the wider lengths of the device enables the treatment of larger coaptation defects. With its narrower design profile, the newly introduced PASCAL Ace Implant System tries to address smaller anatomies and coaptation defects. **Fig. 8** gives an overview of the main characteristics and features of the PASCAL Implant System. Via a 22F transfemoral-venous access route, the delivery system—consisting of a steerable guide sheath, a steerable catheter, and the

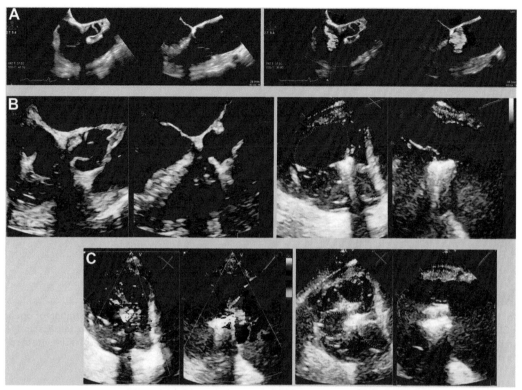

Fig. 6. Edge-to-edge tricuspid valve repair aiming for triple orifice. (*A*) Preinterventional TOE: commissural view (inflow/outflow view) + grasping view ± color Doppler. (*B*) Periinterventional TOE: left, biplane: commissural view + grasping view: deployment/positioning of TriClip XTr; right, biplane: transgastrical view: 1 TriClip XTr anteroseptal deployed, highlighted as a dashed circle: 2 orifices. (*C*) Left: transgastric view + color Doppler: TriClip XTr; right, biplane: transgastric view: triple orifice after deployment of 2 TriClip XTr (anteroseptal and posteroseptal).

implant catheter holding the device—is advanced into the right atrium; in opened position the device is positioned above the tricuspid valve and then inserted into the right ventricle. Slow retraction underneath the leaflets enables the loading of leaflets onto the paddles. Grasping with the clasps can then be obtained either independently or simultaneously. Independent grasping would be advisable in cases of pronounced tethering and/or wider coaptation defects. On close examination of the result with TOE, the device can be reopened, repositioned, and released or retrieved—depending on the result.

The first published case of a successful edge-to-edge treatment of STR with the PASCAL Implant System was reported 2018 by Fam and colleagues in an 82-year-old woman with progressed right heart dilation and failure with torrential TR, edema, and anasarka.[45] The most comprehensive case series so far included 28 patients with ≥severe TR in an observational, non-randomized and single-arm study.[44] All enrolled patients (mean age 78%, 54% female) were highly symptomatic under diuretic medication (89% NYHA Class III, 11% NYHA Class IV; 100% loop diuretics, 68% aldosterone antagonists) and deemed at high surgical risk (EuroSCORE II 6%,2%) by local heart team decision; as expected, the collective presented with multiple comorbidities (eg, 93% atrial fibrillation, 71% renal impairment, 46% coronary artery disease, 18% previous CABG or PCI, respectively). Acute procedural success was 86% with a postprocedural reduction of TR grade to ≤2+ without periprocedural mortality or conversion to open-heart surgery. At 30-day follow-up 15% of patients showed a TR grade ≥3 in comparison to 100% at baseline with corresponding functional improvements in NYHA Class and 6-MWT (incidence of NYHA Class ≥ III at 30-day follow-up: 12% in comparison to 100% at baseline). Moreover, echocardiographic analysis showed a decrease of tricuspid annular dilation from 49 mm ± 8 at baseline to 40 mm ± 7 at follow-up. 1,4 devices were applied per procedure on average—mainly in anteroseptal position (70%, 30% posteroseptal). Two partial device

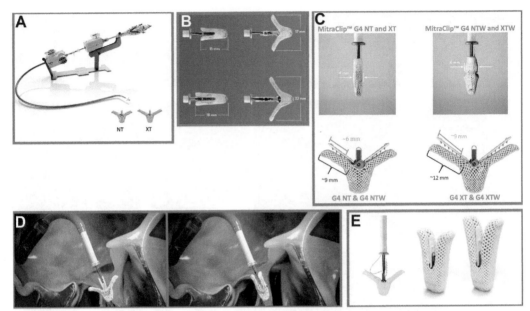

Fig. 7. Main characteristics and features of the TriClip device. (*A*) Delivery system with the illustration of opened TriClip NT and XT. (*B*) Main characteristics and features of TriClipCT XT and NT. (*C*) Main characteristics and features of the MitraClip Generation 4. (*D*) Illustration of leaflet grasping with TriClip. (*E*) Opened TriClip attached to the delivery catheter and TriClip XT and NT in closed configuration.

detachments occurred and 2 deaths within 30 days of follow-up (mortality 7%,1%)—otherwise no short-term complications were observed, suggesting the PASCAL Implant System as a feasible, safe, and effective treatment option for high-risk STR patients.[44] This compassionate use case series led to CE mark in 2020.

In cases of far pronounced right heart dilation, dysfunction, and failure with distinct tricuspid annular dilation and a large coaptation

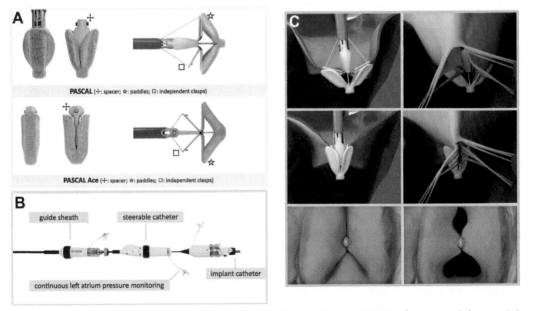

Fig. 8. Main characteristics and features of the PASCAL (Ace) Implant System. (*A*) Main features and characteristics of the PASCAL and PASCAL Ace Implant System. (*B*) Delivery system. (*C*) Illustration of leaflet grasping with PASCAL Implant System.

defect of STR, a combined intervention with direct annuloplasty and subsequent TEER might be promising and has been reported to be safe, feasible and efficient.[46] Moreover, independent grasping of leaflets has proven to be advantageous in cases of profound leaflet tethering and tenting and with wider coaptation defects—in the discussed multicenter compassionate-use trial 90% of patients were treated using independent grasping.[44] However, device maneuvering and navigation and optimal positioning of the larger PASCAL Implant System (in comparison to eg, the TriClip) can be complicated in patients with less dilated right heart cavities and a smaller tricuspid annulus—thus, the smaller PASCAL Ace Implant System was designed to address this difficulty.

Recent propensity-matched analysis could prove the comparable performance of the TriClip device and the PASCAL Implant System in terms of TR reduction, benefit in functional capacity, and mortality; moreover, the incidence of SLDA was similar (5%) for both devices.[47]

Ongoing clinical trials to further analyze the impact of edge-to-edge tricuspid repair are underway (eg, NCT03745313, NCT04614402, NCT04634266). Most importantly, the prospective, randomized-controlled Edwards PASCAL Transcatheter Valve Repair System Pivotal Clinical Trial (CLASP II TR, NCT04097145) evaluates TEER with PASCAL Implant System in comparison to optimal medical therapy (OMT).

Fig. 9 displays an example of TTVr with PASCAL Ace Implant System.

THE CHALLENGES OF SELECTION
Patients–Device–Timepoint of Intervention

After initial diagnosis of symptomatic TR, it is generally recommended, to establish a medical treatment regime first, before initiating further diagnostic tools for procedural planning. Moreover, potentially accompanied left-sided valvulopathies in need of treatment should be addressed first as TR might stabilize or recede afterward. Ideally, the optimal timepoint for intervention should be under compensated conditions with stable symptoms and under optimized heart failure therapy including a sophisticated and individually adjusted diuretic therapy. However, it has to be acknowledged that especially in patients with far progressed (right) heart failure or additional complicating conditions such as renal failure with cardiorenal syndrome or cardiac cirrhosis, a "compensated" state cannot be reached or maintained sometimes, thus, urging further steps toward

(interventional) therapy. Of course, close-meshed clinical and echocardiographic follow-ups are crucial to evaluate disease progression and optimal timing for intervention.

In terms of finding the optimal treatment strategy for each individual patient with symptomatic TR, a detailed evaluation containing TTE, TOE, and cardiac CT is essential and most importantly the discussion in the interdisciplinary heart team.

Various factors have to be taken into account regarding device selection. Of particular consideration in this context is the underlying valvular pathology: in the course of functional TR, annular dilation along the anteroseptal to posteroseptal commissure is common leading to mainly anteroseptal and (less frequently) posteroseptal coaptation defects. In such cases with localized coaptation defects and less advanced annular dilation, leaflet approximation devices are most promising, even though leaflet tethering, tenting, or leaflet (pseudo-) prolapse might complicate the intervention. In contrast, a far progressed and pronounced annular dilation along with significant right ventricular and atrial enlargement with a grave and central coaptation defect makes leaflet approximation devices as a primary approach less promising as the risk of unsuccessful leaflet grasping or an insufficient procedural result is elevated. In this scenario, direct annuloplasty with Cardioband (Edwards Lifesciences, see section 4 of this issue) could serve as a suitable option as a primary approach. If further on results in terms of TR reduction and/or clinical improvement remain unsatisfactory after direct annuloplasty with residual or even recurrent symptomatic TR, case reports showed promising results for subsequent TEER (either in one approach[46] or after reconvalescence)—but this still remains a case-by-case decision.

To select patients who might benefit best from interventional tricuspid valve repair with leaflet approximation devices, predictors for procedural success and failure, respectively, could be identified.[8,29,31,48] for example, a restricted septal leaflet with pronounced tethering and tenting complicates edge-to-edge repair and patients with these pathologies should be carefully selected—in these constellations, independent grasping is a viable option. Moreover, the absence of a central or anteroseptal coaptation defect, a large coaptation gap, a large tenting area, and a large EROA were identified as predictors for procedural failure of edge-to-edge repair with MitraClip and TriClip, respectively—vice versa, a central/

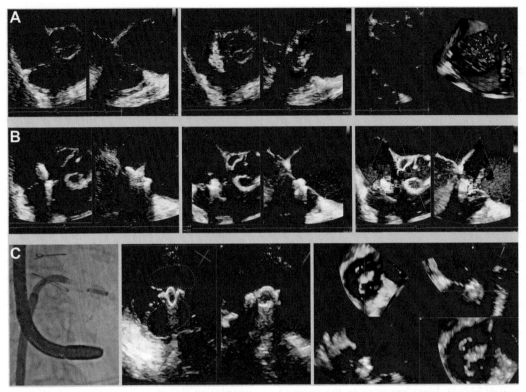

Fig. 9. Edge-to-edge repair with PASCAL Ace Implant System. (A) Preinterventional TOE: left and middle, biplane: commissural view + grasping view ± color Doppler; right: 3D reconstruction of tricuspid valve, highlighted as a dashed circle: coaptation defect. (B) TOE, biplane (commissural view + grasping view): left: deployment/positioning of PASCAL Ace Implant System; middle and right: 1 PA Ace Implant System deployed ± color Doppler. (C) Left: periinterventional fluoroscopy: PASCAL Ace Implant System with delivery catheter and TOE probe; middle, and right: 1 PA Ace Implant System central-anteroseptal with 2 orifices: middle: transgastric view, biplane (highlighted as a dashed circle: 2 orifices); right: 3D reconstructing of the tricuspid valve.

anteroseptal coaptation defect was identified as a predictor for procedural success. Consequently, cut-off margins for exclusion for EROA, tenting area, and gap width were proposed as follows: EROA greater than $0,7$ mm^2, tenting area greater than $3,2$ cm^2, gap greater than $6,4$ mm.[31] Patients beyond these measurements should be referred to and treated in only very experienced centers. Consequently, the risk for SLDA is significantly increased in patients with larger coaptation gaps; for example, the incidence of SLDA in the TRILUMINATE Trial was 7% whereas Braun and colleagues showed an incidence for SLDA of 25% in patients with coaptation gaps >7 mm.[32,49] However, the illustrated iterations of the TriClip device and the larger PASCAL Implant System might address these limitations, nonetheless, conclusive data relating thereto are sparse. Fig. 10 shows an example for SLDA; to stabilize the partially detached device, an additional device can be positioned either in close proximity or opposite (eg,

posteroseptal if SLDA is anteroseptal, Fig. 10 shows an example of the latter).

It must be mentioned, that the proposed interventional procedures require general anesthesia to reduce aspiration risk caused by intraprocedural TOE and to allow for precise device navigation and deployment. In this context, procedural length is an important factor during careful weighting of all device options as patients are often older and multimorbid and general anesthesia has a non-negligible impact on the postprocedural course and outcome. The TRILUMINATE Trial stated a mean procedural time of 153 minutes, the compassionate-use trial for the PASCAL Implant 134 minutes. In contrast, TRI-REPAIR for direct annuloplasty with Cardioband (Edwards Lifesciences, see section 4 of this issue) stated a mean procedural time of 245 minutes, highlighting the different complexities and tolerability of said devices.

Additionally, imaging quality is crucial for procedural success. All of the proposed techniques

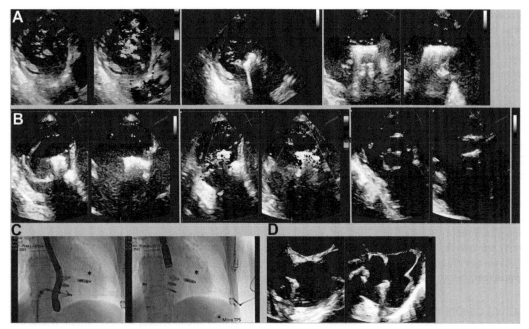

Fig. 10. An Example for single leaflet device attachment (SLDA). (A) TOE, transgastric view: left: preinterventional ± color Doppler; middle: 1 PA Ace Implant System deployed in anteroseptal commissure; right, biplane: 1 additional device in central/posteroseptal position. (B) Transgastric TOE with biplane: left: device anteroseptal in position, SLDA of the device in central/posteroseptal position; right: stabilization with 1 additional Tri-Clip XT posteroseptal. (C) Periinterventional fluoroscopy, left: 2 deployed PASCAL Ace Implant System, 1 TriClip XT in grasping position with the delivery system, Micra TPS, TOE probe; right: 2 deployed PASCAL Ace Implant System, 1 deployed TriClip XT with delivery system retrieved, Micra TPS, TOE probe. (D) TOE, grasping view: additional septum in the right atrium with the delivery system of 1 PA Implant System entangled, also 1 PA Ace Implant System deployed.

require echocardiographic guidance and additional fluoroscopy for precise device navigation and deployment, thus, transoesophageal and transgastric image quality and both imager's and interventionalist's expertise and experience are substantial to ensure optimal results. Artifacts and shadows due to for example, mitral or aortic valve prostheses complicate the procedure and have to be considered. Moreover and regarding the edge-to-edge repair devices (TriClip and PASCAL Implant), their delivery systems and the devices themselves cast artifacts and shadows on the tricuspid valve aggravating echocardiographic visualization and device navigation (the PASCAL Implant System slightly stronger than the TriClip). However, the introduction of 3-dimensional intracardiac echocardiography (ICE) will perspectively enable an additional useful tool in cases of impaired TOE image quality. Moreover, attention should be directed to additional septa in the right atrium, prominent papillary muscles in the right ventricle, or other anatomic variants—both pre- and periinterventionally—as these variants can complicate device navigation and maneuvering. Fig. 10D illustrates an example for device

entanglement in an additional septum in the right atrium.

Additional challenges may arise from ICD- or pacemaker-leads complicating and worsening coaptation defects, TR, and subsequent periprocedural device navigation and deployment. If ICD- or pacemaker-leads are the source or even part of TR etiology, repositioning or extraction before any TR intervention should be evaluated and discussed interdisciplinarily (heart team).

By now, transcatheter tricuspid valve repair has acquired a justified position in line with already established surgical therapy options. So far, the scientific knowledge about said devices indicate a feasible, safe, and efficient treatment option for a growing population of symptomatic patients who would otherwise not be treated beyond optimal heart failure therapy. Patients at high surgical risk or patients with previous heart surgery often get turned down for cardiac surgery, and moreover, combined interventions in high-risk patients with multiple valvulopathies (eg, TAVR for AS plus tricuspid intervention or mitral (TMVR) plus tricuspid intervention) seem beneficial to minimize total procedural time, duration of general anesthesia, time on ICU and in-hospital stay – although tolerability and effectiveness in this context still need further examination as these scenarios to remain case-by-case decisions and adequate data is scarce.

As mentioned above and regarding tricuspid valve repair strategies, renewed, and combined interventions (eg, edge-to-edge-repair following direct annuloplasty) are promising options. Typical indications for this approach include, for example, unsatisfactory TR reduction or recurrence following direct annuloplasty or device detachment (eg, detachment of anchor screws or clip detachment with single-leaflet device attachment, SLDA); but sufficient clinical reports are sparse, these approaches remain case-by-case decisions and belong to the hands of specialized heart centers.

CONCLUSION AND OUTLOOK

ESC Guidelines suggest a class I-recommendation for surgical treatment of refractory severe STR if simultaneous left-sided heart surgery is indicated. Nonetheless, given the fact that the demographic change entails a growing older population at high surgical risk with multiple comorbidities and contraindications for open-heart surgery, there is an increasing need for minimal-invasive and catheter-based treatment options for the equally growing number of patients with STR. In this regard, there are various approaches under clinical development and investigation and early clinical trials investigating TEER and transcatheter direct annuloplasty showed promising outcomes concerning safety, feasibility and efficacy. Randomized and controlled trials with defined endpoints have already started and are mandatory to add crucial long-term follow-up data. Up to now, none of these techniques apply as a gold standard—mainly due to the complex, diverse, and individually variable tricuspid valve anatomy resulting in different shapes and manifestations of subsequent STR. Procedural success critically depends on the optimal timepoint for intervention, careful patient selection, and the choice of the individually most suitable treatment strategy. In this context, pre and periinterventional imaging (mainly TOE and cardiac CT) and thorough procedure planning are of particular importance to ensure a favorable outcome. Current data suggest an even better clinical benefit from TR intervention if TR is treated earlier during the course of the disease—when RV dysfunction and RA and RV dilation still remain less pronounced

and right heart failure symptoms are less prominent. Consequently, there has been a change of strategy during the past decade—notably owing to the growing number of available minimal-invasive treatment options—for the tricuspid valve is no longer called *forgotten*.

CONFLICT OF INTEREST:

J. Vogelhuber: none. M. Weber: MW has received lecture or proctoring fees from Abbott, Boehringer-Ingelheim, Edwards Lifesciences, Janssen, Neochord, Pfizer, and Servier. G. Nickenig: GN has received research funding from the Deutsche Forschungsgemeinschaft, Germany; the German Federal Ministry of Education and Research, Germany; the EU, Abbott, AGA Medical, AstraZeneca, United Kingdom; Bayer, Germany; Berlin Chemie, Biosensus, Biotronic, Bristol-Myers Squibb, United States; Boehringer Ingelheim, Germany; Daiichi-Sankyo, Japan; Edwards Lifesciences, United States; Medtronic, Novartis, Switzerland; Pfizer, United States; Sanofi, United States; and St. Jude Medical, United States; and has received honoraria for lectures or advisory boards from Abbott, AGA Medical, AstraZeneca, Bayer, Berlin, Cardiovalve, Berlin Chemie, Biosensus, Biotronic, Bristol-Myers Squibb, Boehringer Ingelheim, Daiichi Sankyo, Edwards Lifesciences, Medtronic, Novartis, Pfizer, Sanofi, and St Jude Medical.

CLINICS CARE POINTS

- Optimal guideline-directed medical therapy is the backbone of every treatment of symptomatic tricuspid regurgitation.
- Patients with persisting or progressive symptomatic tricuspid regurgitation despite optimized guideline-directed medical therapy should be referred to specialized facilities for further diagnostic and evaluation of individual treatment options.
- Patient-specific treatment recommendations should be discussed by interdisciplinary heart team.

DISCLOSURE

The authors have nothing to disclose.

REFERENCES

1. Prihadi EA. Tricuspid valve regurgitation: no longer the "forgotten valve". ESC E-Journal Cardiol Pract 2018;16.
2. Singh JP, Evans JC, Levy D, et al. Prevalence and clinical determinants of mitral, tricuspid, and aortic regurgitation (the Framingham Heart Study). Am J Cardiol 1999;83(6):897–902.
3. Mangieri A, Pagnesi M, Regazzoli D, et al. Future perspectives in percutaneous treatment of tricuspid regurgitation. Front Cardiovasc Med 2020;7:521211.
4. Benfari G, Antoine C, Miller WL, et al. Excess mortality associated with functional tricuspid regurgitation complicating heart failure with reduced ejection fraction. Circulation 2019;140(3):196–206.
5. Hahn RT. Tricuspid regurgitation: finally unforgettable! Eur Heart J Cardiovasc Imaging 2020;21(2):166–7.
6. Braunwald NS, Ross J Jr, Morrow AG. Conservative management of tricuspid regurgitation in patients undergoing mitral valve replacement. Circulation 1967;35(4 Suppl):I63–9.
7. Essayagh B, Antoine C, Benfari G, et al. Functional tricuspid regurgitation of degenerative mitral valve disease: a crucial determinant of survival. Eur Heart J 2020;41(20):1918–29.
8. Muntane-Carol G, Alperi A, Faroux L, et al. Transcatheter tricuspid valve intervention: coaptation devices. Front Cardiovasc Med 2020;7:139. https://doi.org/10.3389/fcvm.2020.00139.
9. Asmarats L, Taramasso M, Rodes-Cabau J. Tricuspid valve disease: diagnosis, prognosis and management of a rapidly evolving field. Nat Rev Cardiol 2019;16:538–54.
10. Prihadi EA, van der Bijl P, Gursoy E, et al. Development of significant tricuspid regurgitation over time and prognostic implications: new insights into natural history. Eur Heart J 2018;39(39):3574–81.
11. Topilsky Y, Nikomo VT, Vatury O, et al. Clinical outcome of isolated tricuspid regurgitation. JACC Cardiovasc Imaging 2014;7(12):1185–94.
12. Chorin E, Rozenbaum Z, Topilsky Y, et al. Tricuspid regurgitation and long-term clinical outcomes. Eur Heart J Cardiovasc Imaging 2020;21(2):157–65.
13. Yzeiraj E, Bijuklic K, Tiburtius C, et al. Tricuspid regurgitation is a predictor of mortality after percutaneous mitral valve edge-to-edge repair. EuroIntervention 2017;12(15):e1817–24.
14. Schueler R, Ozturk C, Sinning JM, et al. Impact of baseline tricuspid regurgitation on long-term clinical outcomes and survival after interventional edge-to-edge repair for mitral regurgitation. Clin Res Cardiol 2017;106(5):350–8.
15. National Institutes of Health. World's older population grows dramatically. NIH-funded Census Bureau report offers details of global aging phenomenon 2018. Available at: https://www.nih.gov/news-events/news-releases/worlds-older-population-grows-dramatically. Accessed August 18, 2019.
16. Alqahtani F, Berzingi CO, Aljohani S, et al. Contemporary trends in the use and outcomes of surgical treatment of tricuspid regurgitation. J Am Heart Assoc 2017;90:1405–9.
17. Winkel MG, Brugger N, Khalique OK, et al. Imaging and patient selection for transcatheter tricuspid valve interventions. Front Cardiovasc Med 2020;7. Article 60.
18. Holda MK, Zhingre Sanchez JD, Bateman MG, et al. Right atrioventricular valve leaflet morphology redefined: implications for transcatheter repair procedures. JACC Cardiovasc Interv 2019;12(2).
19. Baumgartner H, Falk V, Bax JJ, et al. 2017 ESC/EACTS Guidelines for the management of valvular heart disease. Eur Heart J 2017;38(36):2739–91.
20. Lancellotti P, De Bonis M. Tricuspid regurgitation, in ESC Cardiomed. 3rd edition. Oxford: Oxford University Press; 2019. https://doi.org/10.1093/med/9780198784906.003.0769.
21. Vahanian A, Beyersdorf F, Praz F, et al. 2021 ESC/EACTS Guidelines for the management of valvular heart disease. Eur J Cardiothorac Surg 2021;60(4):727–800. https://doi.org/10.1093/ejcts/ezab389.
22. Taramasso M, Gavazzoni M, Pozzoli A, et al. Tricuspid regurgitation: predicting the need for intervention, procedural success, and recurrence of disease. JACC Cardiovasc Imaging 2019;12(4):605–21. https://doi.org/10.1016/j.jcmg.2018.11.034.
23. Izumi C. Isolated functional tricuspid regurgitation: when should we go to surgical treatment? J Cardiol 2019;75(4):339–43.
24. Hahn RT, Thomas JD, Khalique OK, et al. Imaging assessment of tricuspid regurgitation severity. JACC Cardiovasc Imaging 2019;12(3):469–90.
25. Hashimoto G, Fukui M, Sorajja P, et al. Essential roles for CT and MRI in timing of therapy in tricuspid regurgitation. Prog Cardiovasc Dis 2019;62(6):459–62.
26. Asmarats L, Puri R, Latib A, et al. Transcatheter tricuspid valve interventions: landscape, challenges, and future directions. J Am Coll Cardiol 2018;71(25):2935–56.
27. Curio J, Demir OM, Pagnesi M, et al. Update on the current landscape of transcatheter options for tricuspid regurgitation treatment. Interv Cardiol 2019;14(2):54–61.
28. Latib A, Mangieri A, Agricola E, et al. Percutaneous bicuspidalization of the tricuspid valve using the MitraClip system. Int J Cardiovasc Imaging 2017;33(2):227–8.
29. Lurz P, Besler C, Noack T, et al. Transcatheter treatment of tricuspid regurgitation using edge-to-edge

repair: procedural results, clinical implications and predictors of success. EuroIntervention 2018;14(3): e290–7.

30. Braun D, Orban M, Hagl C, et al. Transcatheter edge-to-edge repair for severe tricuspid regurgitation using the triple-orifice technique versus the bicuspidalization technique. JACC Cardiovasc Interv 2018;11(17):1790–2.

31. Mehr M, Taramasso M, Besler C, et al. 1-year outcomes after edge-to-edge valve repair for symptomatic tricuspid regurgitation: results from the TriValve Registry. JACC Cardiovasc Interv 2019; 12(15):1451–61.

32. Nickenig G, Weber M, Lurz P, et al. Transcatheter edge-to-edge repair for reduction of tricuspid regurgitation: 6-month outcomes of the TRANSIL-LUMINATE single-arm study. Lancet 2019; 394(10213):2002–11.

33. Taramasso M, Gavazzoni M, Pozzoli A, et al. Outcomes of TTVI in patients with pacemaker or defibrillator leads: data from the Trivalve Registry. JACC Cardiovasc Interv 2020;13:554–64.

34. Taramasso M, Hahn RT, Alessandrini H, et al. The international multicenter TriValve registry: which patients are undergoing transcatheter tricuspid repair? JACC Cardiovasc Interv 2017;10(19):1982–90.

35. Mehr M, Kowalski M, Hausleiter J, et al. Combined Tricuspid and mitral versus isolated mitral valve repair for severe mitral and tricuspid regurgitation: an analysis from the TriValve and TRAMI Registries. JACC Cardiovasc Interv 2020.

36. Nickenig G, Kowalski M, Hausleiter J, et al. Transcatheter treatment of severe tricuspid regurgitation with the edge-to-edge MitraClip technique. Circulation 2017;135(19):1802–14.

37. Orban M, Besler C, Braun D, et al. Six-month outcome after transcatheter edge-to-edge repair of severe tricuspid regurgitation in patients with heart failure. Eur J Heart Fail 2018;20(6):1055–62.

38. Taramasso M, Alessandrini H, Latib A, et al. Outcomes after current transcatheter tricuspid valve intervention: mid-term results from the international TriValve registry. JACC Cardiovasc Interv 2019;12(2):155–65.

39. Hahn RT, Zamorano JL. The need for a new tricuspid regurgitation grading scheme. Eur Heart J Cardiovasc Imaging 2017;18(12):1342–3.

40. Lurz P, von Bardeleben RS, Weber M, et al, TRANS-ILLUMINATE Investigators. Transcatheter edge-to-edge repair for treatment of tricuspid regurgitation. J Am Coll Cardiol 2021;77(3):229–39.

41. Corpataux N, Winkel MG, Kassar M, et al. The PASCAL device-early experience with a leaflet approximation device: what are the benefits/limitations compared with the MitraClip? Curr Cardiol Rep 2020;22(8):74.

42. Lim DS, Kar S, Spargias K, et al. Transcatheter valve repair for patients with mitral regurgitation: 30-day results of the CLASP study. JACC Cardiovasc Interv 2019;12(14):1369–78.

43. Praz F, Spargias K, Chrissoheris M, et al. Compassionate use of the PASCAL transcatheter mitral valve repair system for patients with severe mitral regurgitation: a multicentre, prospective, observational, first-in-man study. Lancet 2017;390(10096): 773–80.

44. Fam NP, Braun D, von Bardeleben RS, et al. Compassionate use of the PASCAL transcatheter valve repair system for severe tricuspid regurgitation: a multicenter, observational, first-in-human experience. JACC Cardiovasc Interv 2019;12(24): 2488–95.

45. Fam NP, Ho EC, Zahrani M, et al. Transcatheter tricuspid valve repair with the PASCAL system. JACC Cardiovasc Interv 2018;11(4):407–8.

46. Tabata N, Weber M, Tsujita K, et al. Combined percutaneous therapy for tricuspid regurgitation using the cardioband and PASCAL system in 1 procedure. jACC Cardiovasc Interv 2019;12(22):e197–8.

47. Sugiura A, Vogelhuber J, Öztürk C, et al. PASCAL versus MitraClip-XTR edge-to-edge device for the treatment of tricuspid regurgitation: a propensity-matched analysis. Clin Res Cardiol 2020. https:// doi.org/10.1007/s00392-020-01784-w.

48. Besler C, Orban M, Rommel KP, et al. Predictors of procedural and clinical outcomes in patients with smyptomatic tricuspid regurgitation undergoing transcatheter edge-to-edge repair. JACC Cardiovasc Interv 2018;11:1119–28.

49. Braun D, Rommel KP, Orban M, et al. Acute and short-term results of transcatheter edge-to-edge repair of severe tricuspid regurgitation usig the MitraClip XTR System. JACC Cardiovasc Interv 2019;12:604–5.

Transcatheter Annular Approaches for Tricuspid Regurgitation (Cardioband and Others)

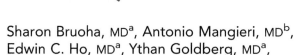

Sharon Bruoha, MD[a], Antonio Mangieri, MD[b],
Edwin C. Ho, MD[a], Ythan Goldberg, MD[a],
Mei Chau, MD[a], Azeem Latib, MD[a],*

KEYWORDS

• Tricuspid regurgitation • Cardioband • Transcatheter tricuspid annuloplasty

KEY POINTS

- Growing evidence supports the independent influence of tricuspid regurgitation (TR) on patient outcomes.
- The postoperative course of isolated tricuspid valve surgery in high-risk patients is associated with poor outcomes.
- Both transcatheter valve replacement and valve repair have emerged as feasible and efficacious, low-risk interventions for TR correction.

INTRODUCTION

The tricuspid valve (TV) often is referred to as "the forgotten valve" because it frequently is managed with only medical therapy due to poor prognostic outcomes with conventional surgical intervention. Nevertheless, a paradigm shift has occurred in recent years, due to a growing evidence base supporting the independent prognostic influence of tricuspid regurgitation (TR) on patient outcomes and the development of lower-risk transcatheter therapies.

Functional TR (FTR), the most prevalent form of TR, seen in approximately 80% of cases, may be a consequence of excessive pulmonary pressure loads (pressure overload) on the right ventricle (RV), causing progressive RV dilatation and dysfunction. Alternatively, long-standing volume overload, as seen in systemic-to-pulmonary shunts, also can induce RV remodeling. RV deformation with subsequent annular dilation and leaflet tethering ultimately lead to FTR. Annular dilatation, typically the dominant mechanism involved in FTR, occurs predominantly along the anteroposterior valve plane, corresponding to the free wall of the RV. Alternatively, in atrial FTR, the right atrium (RA) undergoes progressive dilatation with subsequent annular expansion and leaflet malcoaptation in the absence of pulmonary hypertension (PH).[1,2] Primary TR results from abnormalities of the

Financial Interest: A. Mangieri received an institutional grant from Boston Scientific and is part of the advisory board of Boston Scientific. A. Latib reports the following disclosures: consultant (honoraria)—Edwards Lifesciences, Abbott Vascular; Boston Scientific, Medtronic, Philips, and WL Gore; Scientific Advisory Boards (equity)—Tioga, Supira, NeoChord, CorFlow, and VVital; and Institutional Funding to Montefiore Medical Center from—Edwards Lifesciences, Medtronic, Abbott Vascular, and Boston Scientific.
[a] Department of Cardiology, Montefiore Medical Center, 1825 Eastchester Road, Bronx, NY 10461, USA;
[b] Department of Invasive Cardiology, Humanitas Clinical and Reasearch Center, IRCCS, Via Manzoni, 56, Rozzano, Milan 20089, Italy
* Corresponding author.
E-mail address: alatib@gmail.com

valve leaflets themselves, such as prolapse, flail, perforation, fibrosis, retraction, and congenital abnormalities.

Annular reconstruction frequently is utilized in surgical TV repair. Surgical annular reshaping can be achieved by suture-based or ring-assisted techniques. Suture bicuspidization (Kay procedure) is performed by applying pledget-protected sutures to the posterior annulus with subsequent plication and obliteration of the corresponding segment. Alternatively, surgical annular reduction is performed by the implantation of an undersized, typically incomplete, prosthetic ring. This currently is considered the preferred repair procedure, especially during left-sided valve surgery.[3]

Unfortunately, the postoperative course of isolated TV surgery in high-risk patients, such as redo cardiac surgery, in the presence of severe RV failure, severe PH, or increased surgical risk due to multiple comorbidities, is associated with poor outcomes.[4,5] Therefore, novel transcatheter techniques that replicate surgical annuloplasty are evolving as potentially lower-risk alternatives.

TRICUSPID ANNULAR ANATOMY: IMPLICATIONS FOR THE USE OF PERCUTANEOUS TECHNOLOGIES

The D-shaped tricuspid annulus (TA) is a nonplanar structure and instead has a saddle-shaped 3-dimensional conformation and is devoid of a well-defined annulus fibrosus. The RV free wall attaches to the anterolateral portion of the TA, and the interventricular septum attaches to the relatively shorter septal aspect of the annulus. Histologically, the RV free wall segment contains small amounts of supportive connective tissue whereas the septal segment is in close proximity to the fibrous skeleton of the heart and is more robust. Consequently, annular remodeling is especially pronounced along the axis with less resistance to dilation, along the lateral RV free wall, corresponding to the anteroposterior annulus.

Both transcatheter valve replacement and valve repair have emerged as feasible and efficacious interventions for TR correction. Percutaneous repair techniques that target the leaflets (leaflet-directed) or the TV annulus (annular reshaping therapies) are used most widely and constitute the majority of published evidence.[6]

Effective transcatheter tricuspid repair must overcome multiple potential anatomic obstacles:

- The TV and TA area is dynamic in response to variable loading conditions, positive pressure ventilation, respiratory phase, and cardiac cycle. Thus, the anatomic details obtained during baseline evaluation using transesophageal echocardiography (TEE) or cardiac-gated computed tomography (CT) may differ from the time of intervention. This is due to factors, such as general anesthesia, the supine position of the patient, and intravascular volume status after fasting and preprocedural diuresis, if performed.
- The TV proximity to the right coronary artery (RCA) and conduction system potentially can increase procedure-related risk of iatrogenic injury, causing myocardial ischemia or conduction disease.
- The thin RV free wall is delicate and can be injured or perforated by device manipulation.
- The hinge point of the TV is not demarcated as clearly as in the mitral valve and often is more difficult visualize by TEE due to a lack of fibrous tissue and thick myocardium.
- There often are multiple mechanisms involved in FTR that rarely can be addressed fully using a single repair device. Even if annular dilatation is the predominant mechanism of FTR, associated leaflet coaptation defects, fibrosis, and tethering may result in residual TR despite successful percutaneous annuloplasty. The presence of cardiovascular implantable electronic device (CIED) wires across the TV also may restrict leaflets physically in some situations and reduce the efficacy of annular-directed therapies.[7–10]

IMAGING FOR PATIENT SELECTION AND PROCEDURAL PLANNING

The ideal patients for transcatheter TA reshaping are those with predominantly mild to moderate TA dilatation. Presence of specific disease patterns that may limit the benefit of annular reshaping, therefore, must be evaluated during preprocedural evaluation for appropriate patient selection (Fig. 1):

- Severe leaflet tethering (coaptation depth beyond 10 mm), which occurs as a consequence of advanced RV

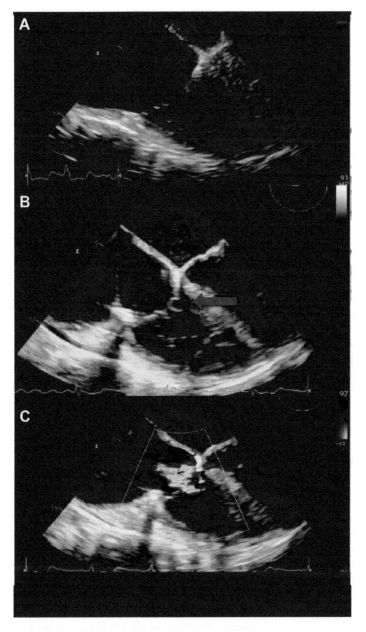

Fig. 1. Example of patient selection considerations for Cardioband (and other annuloplasty devices). TEE images of the TV demonstrating (*A*) annular dilatation with a large coaptation gap and mild leaflet tethering and (*B*) TV septal leaflet tethering (*arrow*) after Cardioband implantation, resulting in (*C*) moderate residual TR.

remodeling, substantially increases annuloplasty failure rates.[11] Annular reshaping techniques effectively stabilize the annular diameter but usually are not sufficient to compensate for leaflet malcoaptation caused by severe leaflet tethering[12] (see **Fig. 1**). A tenting height greater than 0.51 cm and tenting area greater than 0.80 cm^2 also are strong indicators to predict annular reshaping failure, regardless of the device used.[12–14]

- CIED lead-induced TR due to physical constraint of leaflet mobility may not be associated with significant annular dilatation and thus may not benefit as much from annuloplasty alone. In long-standing CIED-lead induced TR, however, annular dilatation frequently is present.
- Primary TR due to severe anatomic leaflet defects cannot be addressed effectively by annuloplasty alone.[15]

- FTR due to severe TA dilatation (>120 mm) may be difficult to treat with transcatheter annular reshaping due to current device size limitations and reduced annular reduction ability in these cases. Patients with large annuli were excluded from some trials.[11,16,17]

If transcatheter annular reshaping is appropriate for a patient's anatomy, it is important to recognize that a standardized anatomic and functional evaluation of the TA for transcatheter TV interventions has been described.[18] Preprocedural evaluation and planning are needed to achieve an optimal result and are based predominantly on echocardiography and cardiac-gated CT.

TA dimensions typically are measured at maximal diastolic opening (end diastole) for optimal device sizing. This can be performed using 3-dimensional TEE or cardiac-gated CT, with CT recognized as the gold standard due to better reproducibility and accuracy. In addition, the evaluation of the anatomic relationship between the RCA and TA is important to understand and minimize the risk of iatrogenic injury during device fixation. This is performed better by CT. Device implantation may be contraindicated if the RCA courses in close proximity to the anchoring site, and there is a high risk of vessel injury.[19,20]

During a procedure, device positioning and implantation typically are guided by real-time TEE, ideally using 3-dimensional techniques, such as multiplanar reconstruction, to optimize anatomic and device visualization. Therefore, evaluation of TEE image quality and windows in the supine position, including the entire TA, is needed before a procedure. Low-quality TEE imaging would hinder a successful and safe procedure substantially if alternative imaging techniques are not available.

THE CARDIOBAND SYSTEM

The Cardioband system (Edwards Lifesciences, Irvine, California) for TV repair, the first Conformité Européenne (CE) mark–approved transcatheter therapy for TR, is a variant of its mitral counterpart (Table 1). It consists of a sutureless contraction band covered by a polyester sleeve that is fixed on the annulus using a series of helical anchors implanted under live imaging guidance along the anterior, lateral, and posterior segments of the TA.

Following implantation, a size-adjustment tool (SAT) facilitates device contraction and annular perimeter reduction. This is performed under live TEE guidance to evaluate the immediate effect of cinching on TR severity. The Cardioband repair system targets the septolateral diameter with a resultant increase in coaptation area between the TV leaflets (Fig. 2) after device deployment.

The Cardioband adjustable annuloplasty system includes 4 main components:

- The implant: consists of a contraction wire covered by a polyester sleeve imprinted with radiopaque markers spaced 8 mm apart. The contraction wire is connected to an adjustment spool that facilitates implant shortening. Implant contraction is performed under live echocardiographic monitoring. Various device sizes are available: 89 mm to 96 mm, 97 mm to 104 mm, 105 mm to 112 mm, and 113 mm to 120 mm; they are matched to the TA size.[11]
- Transfemoral delivery system: the Cardioband delivery system consists of the implant delivery system and the 24F steerable sheath (TSS). The IDS includes a steerable guide catheter and an implant catheter with the Cardioband implant mounted on its distal end.
- Implantable metal anchors and anchor delivery shafts: the Cardioband is fixed to the native TA using 12 to 17 stainless steel helical anchors, deployed in a sequential fashion. The anchors are fully repositionable and retrievable until they are deployed.
- SAT: the SAT distal tip is connected over the implant wire and is used to control the implant adjustment spool and the implant size.

Procedural Steps

After femoral vein access is obtained, the 26F steerable Cardioband sheath is introduced and advanced over a guide wire into the RA. A coronary wire is advanced via arterial access into the RCA to delineate its course and to help demarcate the anterolateral aspect of the annulus on fluoroscopy. This helps facilitate device orientation and implant landing zone localization.

The implant delivery system, consisting of the steerable guide catheter and the implant catheter with the Cardioband device premounted on its distal end, then is introduced to engage the annulus. Band deployment is executed in a stepwise fashion on the atrial side of the annulus in an anterior to posterior, clockwise direction. Initial anchoring at the anteroseptal commissure

Table 1
Transcatheter annuloplasty devices for tricuspid regurgitation repair

Device	Device Type	Description	Current Clinical Experience	Special Considerations
Cardioband system (Edwards Lifesciences, Irvine, CA)	Direct annuloplasty	TA reconstruction via suture-less polyester contraction band delivered and fixated by a series of anchors along the anteroposterior segments of the TA	Clinical trials and real-world data. TRI-REPAIR study (30 patients), US early feasibility study (30 patients), and the international multicenter TriValve registry (13 patients): effective and durable (up to 2 y follow-up) TR reduction and improvement in patients' functional status	Risk of RCA injury
TRAIPTA (National Institutes of Health and Cook Medical, Bloomington, Indiana)	Indirect annuloplasty	The system is introduced in the pericardium through the RA appendage and acts extrinsically at the level of the atrioventricular groove to contract the anterolateral portion of the TA.	Preclinical animal experience showed increases leaflet coaptation.	Challenging procedure with need of pericardial space Risk of coronary injury
TriCinch Coil System (4Tech, Galway, Ireland)	Indirect annuloplasty	The system is secured across the pericardial space using a nitinol coil anchor deployed on the TA (near the anteroposterior commissure) which is connected to a nitinol stent	PREVENT trial (24 patients) showed successful procedure in 85% of patients (2 hemopericardium). Four cases of late anchor detachment	Single anchor with risk of anchor detachment Incomplete plasty with risk of TR recurrence Risk of RCA injury

(continued on next page)

Device	Device Type	Description	Current Clinical Experience	Special Considerations
		placed in the inferior vena cava through a tensioning band.	and 1 case of RCA damage. Currently ongoing early feasibility study in the US (NCT03632967)	
The DaVing TR system (Cardiac Implants, Wilmington, DE)	Direct annuloplasty	Two-stage procedures: ring anchoring to the atrial aspect of the TA favoring tissue healing and a second step of annular size contraction through an adjustment connector fixed to the jugular vein	Currently enrolling for first-in-human study (NCT03700918)	Approximately 90-d interval between procedure stages are required for tissue healing. Risk of RCA injury Risk of atrioventricular block
The Millipede IRIS (Boston Scientific, Marlborough, MA)	Direct annuloplasty	A complete, semirigid, direct annuloplasty nitinol ring delivered to engage the TA with 8 anchors preattached to the base of the implant. Device contraction reduces annular dimensions.	2 patients treated (surgical device implantation): 36% of TA diameter reduction with complete TR abolishment seen immediately after the procedure and sustained for 12 mo. Furthermore, positive remodeling of left ventricle and RV also was noted.	Complete annuloplasty with potential reduced risk for TR recurrence Risk of RCA injury Risk of atrioventricular block

Device	Type	Mechanism	Clinical Data	Advantages/Disadvantages	Image
The MIA-T system (Micro Interventional Devices, PA)	Direct annuloplasty	The annular reduction is achieved without sutures due to the compliant, self-tensioning, MIA implant. Once delivered, traction is applied to anchors, via a connection band, and creates a bicuspidization of the valve by obliterating the posterior leaflet.	STTAR trial (31 patients) showed significant and durable reduction in TA dimensions and TR. No device-related or procedure-related deaths, strokes, or myocardial infarctions reported for any patient throughout the 12-mo follow-up period. The company recently has submitted the required technical documentation for CE mark approval for its MIA-T percutaneous tricuspid annuloplasty system.	Reliable and rapid deployment. Replicate the surgical sutures. Risk of RCA injury. Risk of dehiscence. Limited published data	
Trialign percutaneous TV annuloplasty system (Mitralign, Tewksbury, MA)	Direct annuloplasty	Two pledgets are placed at the anteroposterior and septal-posterior commissures and then cinched together using a plication lock device thus obtaining a plication of the posterior leaflet. Mimics the Kay surgical procedure	Clinical investigations of the Trialign percutaneous TV annuloplasty system were evaluated in 15 patients in SCOUT	Risk of midterm failure (incomplete plasty), which can be mitigated by placing 2 pairs of sutures. Risk of RCA injury	

Abbreviation: TriValve, transcatheter tricuspid valve therapies.

Image of the Davign TR system reproduced with permission from Cardiac Implants LLC, Tarrytown, NY; and Image of the Millipede IRIS provided courtesy of Boston Scientific. © 2021 Boston Scientific Corporation or its affiliates. All rights reserved.

is terminated after posteroseptal commissure, demarcated by the coronary sinus ostium. Up to 17 anchors are utilized to safely secure the device to the annulus, with the number of required anchors corresponding to device size.

Once the Cardioband is anchored to the TA, the size-adjustment tool is introduced over a wire to cinch the implant and reduce the septolateral diameter of the TA. Device anchoring and contraction are monitored carefully by real-time 3-dimensional TEE and fluoroscopy (see **Fig. 2**).[21]

TEE imaging can be challenging during this procedure due to the position of the TA in relation to the esophagus, acoustic shadowing of left-sided implants or calcification, and catheter-associated shadowing of the posterior region of the annulus. In such circumstances, the use of advanced 3-dimensional TEE techniques, such as live multiplanar reconstruction, or alternative modalities, such as intracardiac echocardiography, can help improve visualization of annular hinge points for safe anchor deployment.[17] Finally, fusion imaging combining real-time fluoroscopic and echocardiographic imaging may help facilitate a faster and safer procedure.[21]

Once there is satisfactory restoration of leaflet coaptation and TR reduction, the delivery system is detached and removed from the body.[17]

Early Clinical Results

After early device experience on a compassionate use basis,[22] the safety and the efficacy of the Cardioband implant for the treatment of TR have been evaluated in the TRIcuspid Regurgitation RePAIr With CaRdioband Transcatheter System (TRI-REPAIR) study.[11] Thirty patients with moderate to massive TR (76% had severe to torrential TR) and significant annular septolateral dilatation (>40 mm) who were deemed prohibitive risk for cardiac surgery were enrolled in this single-arm, multicenter, prospective trial.

The Cardioband device was implanted successfully in all patients. At 30 days, 20 of 28 patients (71%) had improved functional status, as assessed by New York Heart Association (NYHA) functional class, to a lower NYHA functional class (P<.0001). At 6 months, patients had a significant improvement of their functional status, as assessed by the Kansas City Cardiomyopathy Questionnaire (KCCQ) score (+24 points

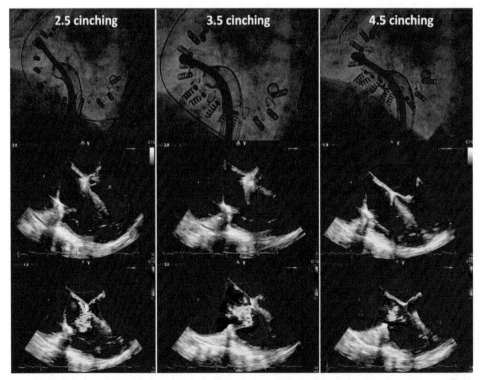

Fig. 2. Cinching of a tricuspid Cardioband with real-time echocardiographic evaluation. Simultaneous fluoroscopy (*top row*) and TEE (*middle* and *bottom rows*) demonstrating sequential degrees of device cinching and associated gradual improvement in septolateral annular diameter and severity of FTR.

change), and the mean 6-minute walk distance increased by 60 m.

The independent core laboratory echocardiographic results reported a significant reduction of the septolateral annular dimensions from 41.6 mm ± 4.9 mm to 36.2 mm ± 4.7 mm (P<.01) at discharge. The reduction remained stable at 30 days (42.2 mm ± 5.1 mm to 37.8 mm ± 3.3 mm; P = .0004) and at 6 months (41.6 mm ± 5.3 mm to 37.8 mm ± 3.4 mm; P = .0014). The effective regurgitant orifice area (EROA) showed a progressive reduction from 0.78 mm^2 ± 0.49 mm^2 at baseline to 0.41 mm^2 ± 0.26 mm^2 at 6 months. Furthermore, only 5 patients (28%) had severe or greater TR at 6 months compared with 14 patients (78%) at baseline (P = .0020).

In light of these positive results, Cardioband has since received the CE mark approval for the treatment of FTR and is being implanted commercially in Europe.

Recently, 2-year follow-up data from the TRI-REPAIR was published.[23] Annular diameter was reduced significantly at discharge and was sustained at 1 year and 2 years. End-diastolic septolateral annular diameter was 41.9 mm ± 4.6 mm (n = 26) at baseline, 36.5 mm ± 3.3 mm (n = 19) at 1 year (P<.001), and 35.2 mm ± 4.6 mm (n = 14) at 2 years (P<.001; paired analysis compared with baseline). Parallel to annular reduction, TR severity improved significantly. Whereas 24% of patients were with less than or equal to moderate TR at baseline, this progressively increased to 63% (P = .007; paired analysis compared with baseline) at 1 year and 72% at 2 years (P = .016; paired analysis compared with baseline). Similarly, the statistically significant reductions in proximal isovelocity surface area (PISA), EROA, and vena contracta (VC) that were seen after the procedure compared to baseline were maintained at 1 year and 2 years.

Functional status also was improved significantly; 17% of patients were classified as NYHA class I–II at baseline, which increased to 78% (P<.001; paired analysis compared with baseline) and 82% (P = .002; paired analysis compared with baseline) at 1 year and 2 years, respectively. In addition, 6-minute walk distance was increased by 42 m at 1 year (P = .053; paired analysis) and 73 m at 2 years (P = .058; paired analysis) compared with baseline. Similarly, the overall KCCQ score was increased by 19 points at 1 year (P<.001; paired analysis) and 14 points at 2 years (P = .046; paired analysis) compared with baseline.

Cardioband experience in the United States also recently was published. A single-arm, multicenter, prospective early feasibility study evaluated the 30-day outcomes of the Cardioband device in 30 patients with symptomatic severe TR despite medical therapy.[17] At baseline, 27% had severe TR, 20% massive TR, and 53% torrential TR. Furthermore, 70% of patients had NYHA functional class III or class IV at enrollment. The device was implanted successfully in 93% of cases. After 30 days, the annular septolateral diameter was reduced by 13% (P<.001) compared with baseline, with associated significant TR reduction and improvement in functional capacity and quality of life. At 1 month, 75% of patients were NYHA functional class I to class II (P<.001). No significant increase in 6-minute walk distance was found. Average reductions of 38% in PISA EROA (0.77 cm^2 vs 0.48 cm^2, respectively; P = .003) and 35% in mean VC (1.4 cm vs 0.9 cm, respectively; P<.001) were seen by echocardiography during the study period. Moreover, indices of RV remodeling, such as mid-RV end-diastolic diameters and RA volume, also were improved significantly 1 month after annular reshaping (Table 2).

Given the promising results thus far, recruitment for the prospective, multicenter Transcatheter Repair of Tricuspid Regurgitation With Cardioband TR System Post-Market Clinical Follow-Up Study (TriBAND) (NCT03779490) currently is ongoing in Europe. The trial is planned to include 150 patients with symptomatic severe FTR who will be treated with the Cardioband system. Device safety and effectiveness will be evaluated during 5 years of follow-up.

Potential Complications

A relatively low rate of complications was reported in the available clinical experience with Cardioband implantation (Table 3).

In TriRepair, 8 deaths occurred during the 2-year follow-up period; 2 cases occurred within the first 30 days (1 was adjudicated as device-related complication). Six deaths that occurred during follow-up were not related to the implant. Two patients underwent device-related secondary interventions as a result of worsening TR. Anchor detachments occurred in 2 patients with subsequent torrential TR.

The investigators reported 3 coronary artery complications: 1 patient had an occlusion of a secondary branch of the RCA, which was left untreated; another patient had worsening of a pre-existing lesion of the distal RCA, which was successfully treated with the implantation of a drug-eluting stent; and 1 patient experienced

Table 2
Changes in echocardiographic and clinical variables between baseline and 30 days

Echocardiographic and clinical variables	TRI-REPAIR			United States Study		
	Baseline	30 Days	P Value	baseline	30 Days	P Value
Echocardiographic variables						
TA septolateral diameter, mm	42.2 ± 0.5	37.8 ± 3.3	.0004	45.4 ± 4.7	39.5 ± 7.4	<.001
PISA EROA, cm²	0.79 ± 0.51	0.39 ± 0.32	.0003	0.84 ± 0.39	0.55 ± 0.41	<.001
Mean VC, cm	1.26 ± 0.45	0.90 ± 0.39	<.0001	1.48 ± 0.48	0.91 ± 0.44	<.001
Mid-RV end-diastolic diameter, cm	3.81 ± 0.62	3.74 ± 0.58	.4943	4.1 ± 0.5	3.7 ± 0.5	<.001
Systolic pulmonary artery pressure, mm Hg	35.8 ± 10.6	39.6 ± 10.7	.0980	37.8 ± 10.9	40.3 ± 12.0	.259
LV ejection fraction, %	57.2 ± 10.5	57.7 ± 8.0	.7664	58.6 ± 5.8	58.5 ± 7.1	.904
LV stroke volume, mL	59.2 ± 19.7	64.5 ± 12.1	0.0716	63.4 ± 16.8	64.1 ± 16.4	.660
Clinical variables						
Severe, massive, or torrential TR, %	71	24	P<.0001	100	56	P<.001
Functional status class NYHA	71% of patients had functional status improvement (NYHA) by 1 or more categories		P<.0001	32% of patients had an NYHA functional status of class I or II	75% of patients had an NYHA functional status of class I or II	P<.001
6MWD, m	261 ± 110	292 ± 123	P = .0759	—	—	Nonsignificant change was reported
KCCQ score	45 ± 23	57 ± 24	P = .0063	53 ± 25	69 ± 24	P<.001

Values are mean ±SD, unless otherwise indicated. The P values were calculated by a Student t test or Wilcoxon signed rank test for paired analyses comparing baseline and 30 d.
Abbreviations: 6MWD, 6-minute walk distance; LV, left ventricular.

Tables 3
Thirty-day adverse events in the Cardioband TRI-REPAIR and early feasibility study in the United States

Adverse Event	TRI-REPAIR No (%)	US Study No (%)
Death	2 (6.7)	0
Stroke	1 (3.3)	0
Myocardial infarction	0	0
Bleeding complications (extensive, life-threatening, or fatal)	4 (13.3)	7 (23.3)
Coronary complications	3 (10.0)	1 (3.3)
Anchor detachment	0	2 (6.7)
Device-related secondary intervention	0	0
Device-related cardiac surgery	0	0
Conduction system disturbance	1 (3.3)	0
Ventricular arrhythmia	2 (6.7)	0

pericardial tamponade secondary to penetration of 1 anchor into the successfully CA. The perforation was managed successfully with prolonged balloon inflation and pericardial drainage. This complication potentially can be mitigated with the use of advanced echocardiographic techniques, such as live 3-dimensional multiplanar reconstruction and echocardiographic-fluoroscopic fusion to better visualize the anchor implant zone. In the early feasibility trial performed in the United States, 1 episode of iatrogenic RCA deformation that was treated with 2 drug-eluting stents.

Iatrogenic RCA deformations were evaluated in a recent analysis of 51 patients treated with Cardioband. RCA distortion was evident in 14 of 51 (36.5%) implantations. In 12 cases, although angiographically severe (estimated visually as ≥80% stenosis), no flow impairment or signs of dissection, perforation, or occlusion were observed. Moreover, no signs of ischemia were evident on electrocardiography and no biochemical markers of myocardial injury were evident. A conservative approach was chosen and follow-up angiography (mean of 5.36 days ± 7.73 days after implantation) revealed complete reversal of RCA abnormalities, whereas 2 deformations were treated by stenting.[20] Thus, postimplantation lesions without flow limitations associated with Cardioband implantation often are self-resolving over time and can be managed conservatively if there is no clear indication for immediate stent implantation.

Periprocedural bleeding occurred in 4 patients (13.3%) in the TRI-REPAIR and 7 patients (23.3%) in the early feasibility US study. Two

patients, 1 in each study, developed cardiac tamponade during the procedure. In TRI-REPAIR, 1 fatal case of subarachnoid hemorrhage was reported.

OTHER TRANSCATHETER TRICUSPID ANNULOPLASTY SYSTEMS

There currently are several transcatheter devices, which aim to replicate complete or incomplete surgical tricuspid annuloplasty that are in the preclinical or clinical investigational phase of development (see Table 1)

Transatrial Intrapericardial Tricuspid Annuloplasty

The transatrial intrapericardial tricuspid annuloplasty (TRAIPTA) (National Institutes of Health and Cook Medical, Bloomington, Indiana) is an indirect annuloplasty system delivered through the pericardial space and across the atrioventricular groove. The system is introduced in the pericardium through the right appendage to externally reduce the anterolateral portion of the TA. The system has been tested in 16 Yorkshire swine with successful delivery in all cases without complications. Implantation resulted in a reduction of annular dimensions, annular perimeter and TV area. In 4 animal models with baseline TR, TRAIPTA achieved a significant and stable reduction of the insufficiency.[24] The first-in-human implantation is pending.

TriCinch

The TriCinch Coil System (4Tech Cardio, Galway, Ireland) is an indirect annuloplasty device in its second generation. Contrary to the first-generation device, which was anchored directly to the hinge point of the lateral TA using a corkscrew-shaped anchor, the second-generation device is secured in the pericardial space using a nitinol coil with a hemostasis seal anchor. This anchor is connected to a nitinol stent placed in the inferior vein cava through a tensioning band, which pulls the lateral annulus toward the septum. These modifications to the second-generation device were designed to overcome the main limitation of the previous Tri-Cinch system, that is, dehiscence and loss of efficacy.

In the Percutaneous Treatment of Tricuspid Valve Regurgitation With the TriCinch System (PREVENT) trial (NCT02098200), implantation of the first-generation TriCinch was successful in 18 cases and a reduction of TR by at least 1 grade occurred in 94% of the cases. Two patients had hemopericardium after the procedure and late detachment of the corkscrew shaped anchor was observed in 4 patients.[8]

After 2 successful procedures in the United States and many in Europe, the TriCinch coil system is under investigation in the Early Feasibility Study of the Percutaneous 4Tech TriCinch Coil Tricuspid Valve Repair System (NCT03632967). This study aims to treat patients with at least moderate TR in 7 centers across the United States.[25] Device development since has been interrupted because of financial reasons.

DaVingi
The DaVingi TR system (Cardiac Implants, Wilmington, Delaware) is a transcatheter tricuspid annuloplasty system that is implanted in a 2-step procedure. The device is first delivered through a 22F catheter from the jugular vein and positioned on the atrial aspect of the TA. It is fixed to the annulus by simultaneously firing a set of anchors. The presence of a prosthesis ring favors a healing process so that, in a second step procedure done approximately 3 months later, the annular size is adjusted through an adjustment connector fixed to the jugular vein. The first 5 patients of a first-in-human study have been enrolled (NCT03700918).[8]

Millipede IRIS
The Millipede IRIS device (Boston Scientific, Marlborough, Massachusetts) is a complete, semirigid, nitinol ring that is attached to the TA with 8 helical anchors that are preattached to the base of the implant. It functions as a direct annuloplasty device. The upper portion of the device has 8 sliding collars, which, when advanced, decreases the distance between 2 adjacent anchoring elements. Each ring segment (consisting of 1 sliding collar and 2 anchors) can be adjusted independently, allowing selective remodeling of the most dilated portions of the annulus. The ring is completely retrievable for optimal repositioning prior to deployment. The 3 basic steps of the Millipede IRIS procedure are (1) placement, (2) anchoring, and (3) adjustment.[8,26]

The Millipede IRIS has been implanted during open heart surgery as proof-of-concept in 3 patients during a combined procedure to treat both TR and MR. After placement and anchoring, the collars were advanced to reduce the size of the device and attached annulus until leaflet coaptation was achieved and there was no TR by surgical bulb testing.

Significant reduction in TR to trace was noted, with an average TA septolateral diameter reduction of 36% that was stable at 6-month and 12-month follow-up. A dedicated delivery catheter for transcatheter deployment to the TA is under development.[26]

MIA-T System
The MIA-T system (Micro Interventional Devices, Newtown, Pennsylvania) consists of a series of low-mass, polymeric, self-tensioning PolyCor anchors and a thermoplastic elastomer, MyoLast, for tensioning of the anchors inducing annular plication. A dedicated 12F delivery catheter is used for anchor deployment. Once delivered, the anchors are linked using a connection band, which then is tightened to bicuspidize the valve by obliterating the posterior leaflet. A total of 31 patients supposedly have been enrolled thus far in the percutaneous arm of the Study of Transcatheter Tricuspid Annular Repair (STTAR) trial (NCT03692598). The company has reported significant reductions in annular dimensions and TR with MIA-T system and durable results at 1-year follow-up. There are no published data, however, on these patients. The company recently has submitted the required technical documentation for CE mark approval based on these data.[8]

Trialign
The Trialign percutaneous TV annuloplasty system (Mitralign, Tewksbury, Massachusetts) is a transcatheter incomplete direct annuloplasty system designed to mimic the Kay surgical procedure. Using a transjugular approach, 2 pledgets are placed at the anteroposterior and posterior-septal commissures, followed by cinching using a plication lock device to eliminate the posterior leaflet to bicuspidize the valve. The performance of the device has been tested in the

Percutaneous Tricuspid Valve Annuloplasty System for Symptomatic Chronic Functional Tricuspid Regurgitation (SCOUT) I and SCOUT II trial.[27] Device development has since been interrupted because of financial reasons.

SUMMARY

Transcatheter tricuspid interventions are progressively gaining importance in the undertreated TR patient population, especially in the setting of those at high surgical risk. Several devices aiming to achieve TA remodeling, by direct or indirect annuloplasty, have been designed to treat 1 of the primary mechanisms for FTR. These devices require specific preprocedural assessment to ensure appropriate patient selection and to maximize the likelihood of success by designing through careful procedural planning. Because many of these devices still are in the early stages of development, further experience with larger cohorts of patients are under way to better evaluate procedural and clinical outcomes.

CLINICS CARE POINTS

- FTR is the most prevalent form of TR, arising in the setting of RV remodeling.
- Severe TR is associated with poor patient outcomes.
- Available drug therapy specific for TR is highly limited and is based mainly on diuretics. Treating the underlying etiologies associated with secondary TR is strongly recommended.
- Surgical annuloplasty currently is considered the preferred repair procedure, especially during left-sided valve surgery.
- Surgical repair of isolated TR in high-risk patients with evidence of end-organ damage is associated with poor outcomes. Thus, treatment should be pursued early, before the onset of severe PH and/or severe RV failure.
- Novel transcatheter techniques that replicate surgical annuloplasty are evolving as effective and lower-risk alternatives.

REFERENCES

1. Dreyfus GD, Martin RP, Chan KM, et al. Functional tricuspid regurgitation: a need to revise our understanding. J Am Coll Cardiol 2015;65(21):2331–6.

2. Sanz J, Sánchez-Quintana D, Bossone E, et al. Anatomy, function, and dysfunction of the right ventricle: JACC state-of-the-art review. J Am Coll Cardiol 2019;73(12):1463–82.

3. Rausch MK, Bothe W, Kvitting JP, et al. Mitral valve annuloplasty: a quantitative clinical and mechanical comparison of different annuloplasty devices. Ann Biomed Eng 2012;40(3):750–61.

4. Saran N, Dearani JA, Said SM, et al. Long-term outcomes of patients undergoing tricuspid valve surgery†. Eur J Cardiothorac Surg 2019;56(5):950–8.

5. Subbotina I, Girdauskas E, Bernhardt AM, et al. Comparison of outcomes of tricuspid valve surgery in patients with reduced and normal right ventricular function. Thorac Cardiovasc Surg 2017;65(8): 617–25.

6. Santaló-Corcoy M, Asmarats L, Li CH, et al. Catheter-based treatment of tricuspid regurgitation: state of the art. Ann Transl Med 2020;8(15):964.

7. Topilsky Y, Khanna AD, Oh JK, et al. Preoperative factors associated with adverse outcome after tricuspid valve replacement. Circulation 2011; 123(18):1929–39.

8. Curio J, Demir OM, Pagnesi M, et al. Update on the current landscape of transcatheter options for tricuspid regurgitation treatment. Interv Cardiol 2019;14(2):54–61.

9. Dahou A, Levin D, Reisman M, et al. Anatomy and physiology of the tricuspid valve. JACC Cardiovasc Imaging 2019;12(3):458–68.

10. Besler C, Orban M, Rommel KP, et al. Predictors of procedural and clinical outcomes in patients with symptomatic tricuspid regurgitation undergoing transcatheter edge-to-edge repair. JACC Cardiovasc Interv 2018;11(12):1119–28.

11. Nickenig G, Weber M, Schueler R, et al. 6-month outcomes of tricuspid valve reconstruction for patients with severe tricuspid regurgitation. J Am Coll Cardiol 2019;73(15):1905–15.

12. Fukuda S, Song JM, Gillinov AM, et al. Tricuspid valve tethering predicts residual tricuspid regurgitation after tricuspid annuloplasty. Circulation 2005;111(8):975–9.

13. Taramasso M, Alessandrini H, Latib A, et al. Outcomes after current transcatheter tricuspid valve intervention: mid-term results from the international TriValve registry. JACC Cardiovasc Interv 2019;12(2):155–65.

14. Taramasso M, Hahn RT, Alessandrini H, et al. The international multicenter TriValve registry: which patients are undergoing transcatheter tricuspid repair? JACC Cardiovasc Interv 2017;10(19):1982–90.

15. Fukuda S, Gillinov AM, McCarthy PM, et al. Determinants of recurrent or residual functional tricuspid regurgitation after tricuspid annuloplasty. Circulation 2006;114(1 Suppl):I582–7.

16. Tornos Mas P, Rodríguez-Palomares JF, Antunes MJ. Secondary tricuspid valve regurgitation: a forgotten entity. Heart 2015;101(22):1840–8.

17. Davidson CJ, Lim DS, Smith RL, et al. Early feasibility study of cardioband tricuspid system for functional tricuspid regurgitation: 30-day outcomes. JACC Cardiovasc Interv 2021;14(1):41–50.

18. Ro R, Tang GHL, Seetharam K, et al. Echocardiographic imaging for transcatheter tricuspid edge-to-edge repair. J Am Heart Assoc 2020;9(5): e015682.

19. Schueler R, Hammerstingl C, Werner N, et al. Interventional direct annuloplasty for functional tricuspid regurgitation. JACC Cardiovasc Interv 2017;10(4):415–6.

20. Gerçek M, Rudolph V, Arnold M, et al. Transient acute right coronary artery deformation during transcatheter interventional tricuspid repair with the Cardioband tricuspid system. EuroIntervention 2021;17(1):81–7.

21. Pascual I, Pozzoli A, Taramasso M, et al. Fusion imaging for transcatheter mitral and tricuspid interventions. Ann Transl Med 2020;8(15):965.

22. Kuwata S, Taramasso M, Nietlispach F, et al. Transcatheter tricuspid valve repair toward a surgical standard: first-in-man report of direct annuloplasty with a cardioband device to treat severe functional tricuspid regurgitation. Eur Heart J 2017;38(16):1261.

23. Nickenig G, Weber M, Schüler R, et al. Tricuspid valve repair with the Cardioband system: two-year outcomes of the multicentre, prospective TRI-REPAIR study. EuroIntervention 2020;16(15): e1264–71.

24. Rogers T, Ratnayaka K, Sonmez M, et al. Transatrial intrapericardial tricuspid annuloplasty. JACC Cardiovasc Interv 2015;8(3):483–91.

25. Rodés-Cabau J, Taramasso M, O'Gara PT. Diagnosis and treatment of tricuspid valve disease: current and future perspectives. Lancet 2016; 388(10058):2431–42.

26. Rogers JH, Boyd WD, Bolling SF. Tricuspid annuloplasty with the Millipede ring. Prog Cardiovasc Dis 2019;62(6):486–7.

27. Hahn RT, Meduri CU, Davidson CJ, et al. Early feasibility study of a transcatheter tricuspid valve annuloplasty: SCOUT trial 30-day results. J Am Coll Cardiol 2017;69(14):1795–806.

Transcatheter Tricuspid Valve Replacement for Surgical Failures

Marvin H. Eng, MD[a],*, Pradeep Yadav, MD[b],
Vinod Thourani, MD[c], Kenith Fang, MD[d]

KEYWORDS

- Transcatheter • Tricuspid valve replacement • Tricuspid surgery • Tricuspid repair

---

KEY POINTS

- Reoperation for failed tricuspid repairs or replacements is fraught with excessive mortality rates.
- Tricuspid valve-in-valve (TViV) is relatively straight forward with reasonable intermediate-term results.
- Tricuspid valve-in-ring (TVIR) has higher risks of valve malpositioning, valve embolization, and paravalvular leak. These cases should be approached with more caution.
- Predictors of mortality include age and decompensated clinical status before transcatheter intervention.

INTRODUCTION

Transcatheter valve therapy has ushered an era of percutaneous treatment of especially ill or complex patients. Patient with failed surgical tricuspid valve repairs or replacements are especially vulnerable and initial treatment with percutaneous valve seems to be a promising treatment.[1–3]

Approximately 5400 tricuspid valve surgeries occur in the United States annually, of which 89% are repairs.[4] The 15-year freedom from reoperation for bioprosthetic valves is 55.1 ± 13.8% and the reoperation rate estimates to be 2.68% per year.[5] And for most of the patients undergoing tricuspid valve repair, 13% to 14% of repairs have 3 to 4+ tricuspid regurgitation postoperatively.[6,7] Operative mortality for first-time tricuspid valve surgery is already elevated at 10.6%, and retrospective data indicate that reoperation for TR is fraught with even higher mortality.[8,9] Society of thoracic surgery (STS) noted that

first reoperation for tricuspid valve surgery demonstrates a 1.7 odds[4] for 30-day mortality and retrospective registries have documented a 22% to 37% mortality rate.[6,9,10]

With a clear need for an alternative to redo surgery, transcatheter heart valve (THV) implantation presents itself as a tangible option. The first report of a tricuspid valve replacement was within a cohort of patients that underwent valve-in-valve (ViV) in all 4 positions,[1] and then several retrospective registries or case series have been published.[11–13]

The largest experience published thus far exists in the ViV international database (VIVID).[11,12] The VIVID registry found that 59% of transcatheter valve replacements were for patients with congenital heart disease. The remainder of patients with acquired heart disease includes patients with endocarditis, rheumatic heart disease, functional tricuspid regurgitation, and tricuspid valve injury related to biopsies and trauma. Median number

---

[a] Division of Cardiology, Structural Heart Program, University of Arizona, Banner University Medical Center, 1111 East McDowell Road, Phoenix, AZ 85006, USA; [b] Division of Cardiology, Piedmont Heart Institute, 275 Collier Road Northwest #500, Atlanta, GA 30309, USA; [c] Division of Cardiothoracic Surgery, Piedmont Heart Institute, 275 Collier Road Northwest #500, Atlanta, GA 30309, USA; [d] Division of Cardiothoracic Surgery, Banner University Medical Center, 1111 East McDowell Road, Phoenix, AZ 85006, USA
* Corresponding author.
E-mail address: marvin.eng@bannerhealth.com

Intervent Cardiol Clin 11 (2022) 81–86
https://doi.org/10.1016/j.iccl.2021.09.008
2211-7458/22/© 2021 Elsevier Inc. All rights reserved.

of prior surgeries was 2 (range 1–10). It seems that most patients undergoing the therapy have degenerated valves (93%) and the majority have atrial fibrillation (44%).[12]

PROCEDURAL CONSIDERATIONS
Transcatheter Heart Valve Choice
Balloon-expandable valves have been the only type of prosthesis used for transcatheter tricuspid valve replacement (TTVR). The 2 prosthesis types used have been the Melody (Medtronic, Minneapolis, MN) and Edwards Sapien (Edwards Lifesciences, Irvine, CA) valve series.

Melody Transcatheter Heart Valve
The Melody valve is composed of bovine jugular vein mounted onto a gold welded platinum-iridium frame. It is available in 2 sizes 16 mm and 18 mm and comes with the Ensemble and Ensemble II delivery system. Medtronic instructions for use (IFU)[14] for the valve and delivery system dimensions are as listed in Tables 1 and 2, respectively. The bovine jugular vein is specifically used for low-pressure systems, specifically right heart pressures, and the manufacturer recommends against using the THV in the mitral or aortic position. As noted in Table 2, the valve delivery system has a smaller balloon within a larger balloon, better known as a balloon-in-balloon (BiB) system and as such, uses a 2-step inflation. The delivery sheath size required is 22 French (Fr).[14]

Edwards Sapien Series
The Edwards Sapien valve is a bovine pericardial valve mounted onto a cobalt-chromium frame. There are 3 iterations: the Sapien 3000 TFX, Sapien XT, and Sapien 3. The newest version of the Sapien 3 includes an additional PTFE skirt on the exterior of the base of the valve designed to minimize paravalvular leaks. The Sapien 3 is manufactured in 4 sizes: 20 mm, 23 mm, 26 mm, and 29 mm. Due to the typical size of bioprosthetic valves and annuloplasty rings in adult cardiac patients, we anticipate using 29 mm Sapien 3 Valve for most noncongenital patients. The Sapien 3 is delivered via a 14-16 Fr expandable or a 22-24 Fr non-expandable sheath.

PROCEDURE TECHNIQUE
Vascular Access
The usual routes of delivery for performing transcatheter tricuspid ViV or ViR are either the transfemoral or the internal jugular route (Fig. 1). In theory, the axillary/subclavian vein is a possible but seldom used access for this procedure. The path from the internal jugular path provides coaxial alignment with the disadvantage of increased operator radiation exposure. Transfemoral route has the advantage of mimicking the haptics of routine procedures in the catheterization laboratory but coaxial alignment is more variable. Features influencing coaxial alignment from the transfemoral route include: right ventricular (RV) depth, inferior vena cava (IVC) and RV angle, IVC tortuosity and the presence of prominent Eustachian valves or Chiari networks may influence valve delivery from the femoral route.

Implantation Within a Degenerative Valve Prosthesis
In the largest experience from the VIVID registry, approximately half of the patients have pure regurgitation, one-fourth of the patients pure stenosis, and the remaining mixed stenosis and regurgitation.[15] THV implantation within a degenerated prosthesis is more forgiving due to the presence of posts to assist with THV alignment. The posts of the prosthesis can range from 12 to 26 mm depending on the size and manufacturer of the valve.[16] The presence of posts and their ability to help orient the THV allows for some flexibility for coaxial alignment and enables secure implantation despite imperfect coaxial alignment. Some of the bioprostheses have minimally radiopaque sewing rings, such as the Biocor Epic valve (Abbott Vascular, Santa Clara, CA), and may be challenging to visualize.

Suboptimal THV expansion or elevated residual gradients have prompted bioprosthetic valve fracture.[17] Generally, high-pressure inflation is required with a noncompliant balloon (True balloon or Vida, Bard Medical, Covington, GA). There are no clear guidelines for balloon sizing relative to the bioprosthetic valve as the current guideline published is for aortic bioprosthetic fracture and the recommendation is 1 mm higher than the manufacturer labeled prosthesis diameter. Give the proximity of the right coronary artery to the tricuspid annulus, we recommend caution with bioprosthetic fracture. Pressures as high as 20 ATM have been used to achieve success. There is scant information about the long-term effects of high-pressure inflations on bioprosthetic leaflet function; therefore, the role of fracturing should be reserved

Table 1
Melody valve size and maximal dimensions per Medtronic instructions for use (IFU)

Melody Valve	Maximal Diameter (IFU)
16 mm	20 mm
18 mm	22 mm

Table 2
Medtronic Ensemble delivery catheter recommended delivery pressures and maximal dimensions

Delivery System Size Inner/Outer Balloon	Inner Balloon Rated Burst Pressure ATM	Outer Balloon Rated Burst Pressure ATM	Resulting Valve Outer Diameter mm
18 mm 9mm × 3.5 cm/18 mm × 4 cm	5	4	20.1
20 mm 10 mm × 3.5 cm/20 mm × 4 cm	5	4	22.4
22 mm 11 mm × 3.5 cm/22 mm × 4 cm	4.5	3	24.1

Abbreviation: ATM, atmospheres.

for underexpanded THV's or high residual gradients. Higher residual gradient post-TTVR was associated with shorter freedom from reintervention (HR 1.14 per mm Hg, $P = .0005$) and should be addressed in the index transcatheter procedure if possible.[12]

Failed Tricuspid Valve Repairs and Tricuspid Valve-In-Ring

Implantation within degenerated annuloplasty rings is more challenging and fraught with more risk of valve malpositioning, embolization, or paravalvular leak. Annuloplasty rings used in the tricuspid position are frequently incomplete and resemble a spiral staircase, thus posting a challenge to sealing (Fig. 2).[13] Although the manufacturer has standard sizes for the annuloplasty rings, remodeling, and progressive annular dilation may distort ring dimensions. A thorough analysis with echocardiography and computed tomography (CT) imaging should be performed to better understand the dimensions of the annuloplasty ring, presence of ring dehiscence, and to gain some understanding of the risk of paravalvular leak.

Coaxial alignment is a top priority for TVIR due to the short landing zone. Of note, some procedures did have prevalve stenting in a small registry to facilitate valve implantation.[13] Valve malalignment should not be accepted and an alternative access route should be used if initial valve delivery appears noncoaxial. Confirmatory balloon sizing was performed in about half the registry cases and is recommended when there is concern that the THV could be undersized.

TTVIR procedures occur seldomly, the VIVD registry analysis showed only 7% of cases implanted within annuloplasty rings.[12] A small, multicenter retrospective series found a 15% rate of procedural complications.[13] Significant paravalvular leak was common (30%) and there was one valve embolization. One repeat TVIR was performed for severe regurgitation. Relevant skills for treating paravalvular leaks are a prerequisite for performing TVIR. The leaks are most frequently at the medial side near the septum as most incomplete rings orient the noncontiguous portion of the annuloplasty ring toward the septum.

Management of Pacing and Pacemakers During Transcatheter Tricuspid Valve Replacement

Usually, it is unnecessary to perform rapid pacing when implanting in the tricuspid position. However, if the patient does have elevated RV systolic pressure of the operators insist on rapid pacing during implantation, then they can choose between using an already present pacemaker lead, pacing from a coronary vessel, or

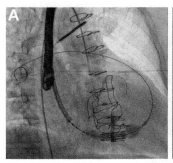 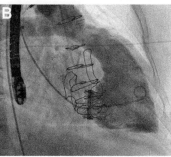

Fig. 1. Transjugular approach to transcatheter tricuspid valve replacement. (A) Right internal jugular provides excellent coaxial alignment to a prosthesis in the tricuspid position. (B) Postright ventriculography demonstrates no regurgitation postvalve implantation.

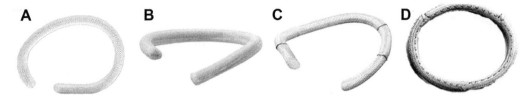

Fig. 2. Commercially available tricuspid annuloplasty rings. Note that most are not planar in configuration and have a 3-dimensional shape. (A) Carpentier-Edwards Classic; (B) Carpentier Edwards MC3; (C) Medtronic Contour; (D) Medtronic Sculptor. (Figure is adapted from Aboulhosn, J et al. JACC: Cardiovascular Interventions 2017;10:53–63, permissions granted).

attempt to use the THV delivery wire for pacing.[18] Of note, rapid pacing was used 22% of the time in the VIVID registry patients.[12]

Of 329 patients analyzed in the VIVID registry, 31 patients underwent valve implantation across a transvenous pacing lead. In this subcohort, 3.2% and 6.4% suffered RV lead dislodgement and RV lead failure respectively. Therefore, THV implantation across pacing leads is possible with a small rate of pacing-related complications.[15] Although 2 patients did have preemptive lead extraction with reimplantation, this seems unnecessary. Should operators proceed with THV implantation across the pacing lead, there should be preparatory arrangements made for possible pacemaker lead revision immediately following valve implantation. Consideration should be made for either leadless or coronary sinus lead implantation to avoid jeopardizing the competency of the new THV. Moreover, repeat assessment of lead function and integrity should be performed before discharge and during follow-up.

Tricuspid Valve Reintervention

A total of 10% of patients required TV reintervention during the follow-up period. Surgical TVR was performed in 18 patients, 2nd TTVR was performed in 8 patients. Reasons for repeat intervention are listed in Box 1.

Durability

Only intermediate follow-up data are available at this time. The VIVID registry showed that 14/306 patients were found to have significant valve dysfunction at 15.8 months.[12] Antithrombotic use and post-THV valve dysfunction did not directly correlate, 32% of patients with post-THV regurgitation or stenosis were prescribed antithrombic agents as compared 52% of patients without valve dysfunction. Determinants of valve durability include formation of thrombus and endocarditis but there was no mention of pannus formation in the reports.

Valve Thrombosis: A total of 8 patients suffered valve thrombosis ranging from a few days post-TTVR to 6-months postvalve implantation. Some cases did resolve with anticoagulation; however, 2 patients did eventually require surgery. The incidence of thrombosis was 0.033 at 3 years and elevated postprocedural gradients were an independent risk factor for valve thrombosis (HR 1.38 per mm Hg, $P = .002$). Post-THV anticoagulation safety data are scant, we can only extrapolate from mechanical tricuspid prosthesis data where rates of gastrointestinal and intracranial bleeding were 16% and 5% respectively.[9] Currently we recommend that patients be treated with anticoagulation post-TTVR indefinitely if possible and patients intolerant to anticoagulation be considered for an alternative to TTVR.

Endocarditis

Eight patients were diagnosed with endocarditis post-THV.[12] Incidence of endocarditis was 0.017 at 1 year and 0.042 at 3 years. The annualized incidence rate was calculated to be 1.5% per patient-year. Of the endocarditis patients, 3 were treated with surgery and 4 with medical therapy. No deaths resulted from endocarditis.

Survival: Median follow-up was 15.9 months. Early death was rare, 2.6% died within 30 days. Multivariate analysis showed that the acute illness/recent hospitalization (HR 4.4, $P < .001$) and older age (HR 1.03 per year, $P < .001$) as

| Box 1 |
Indications for TV Reintervention after TTVR
Transcatheter heart valve dysfunction
Paravalvular leak
Endocarditis
Valve thrombosis
Concurrent intervention (i.e. heart transplantation)
Acute valve embolization
Persistent multiorgan failure with suspected tricuspid dysfunction

independent predictors for mortality. Cumulative incidence of death was 0.18.[12]

SUMMARY

Percutaneous TTVR for failed tricuspid surgeries is similar to the experience in the mitral valve whereby ViV procedures are more reproducible than ViR procedures. TViV is not particularly technically challenging and has consistently good results with few procedural complications. However TViR is difficult due to the anatomic nature of tricuspid annuloplasty rings/bands thus resulting in higher rates of valve malposition and paravalvular leak. As future orthotopic valve replacements are clinically developed, TTVR for failed tricuspid repairs may use orthotopic valves rather than off-label use of balloon-expandable valves. Future investigations will need to assess for THV durability and thromboprophylaxis duration in the tricuspid position. TTVR for surgical failures is currently relatively rare, but with the more aggressive stance of tricuspid valve surgical repairs, we should expect to encounter this challenge more frequently in the near future.

DISCLOSURES

Marvin H. Eng, MD is a clinical proctor for Edwards Lifesciences and Medtronic.

CLINICS CARE POINTS

- Transcatheter Tricuspid Valve Replacement (TTVR) is a feasible alternative to repeat surgery for failed tricuspid surgical valves or repairs.
- Tricuspid Valve-in-Ring is more complex and nuance than Tricuspid Valve-in-Valve due anatomic nature of incomplete tricuspid rings/bands.
- Decompensated patient clinical status is an independent risk factor for mortality in TTVR cases.
- Elevated post-TTVR gradients are predictors of repeat intervention.

REFERENCES

1. Webb JG, Wood DA, Ye J, et al. Transcatheter valve-in-valve implantation for failed bioprosthetic heart valves. Circulation 2010;121:1848–57.
2. Ruparelia N, Mangieri A, Ancona M, et al. Percutaneous transcatheter treatment for tricuspid bioprosthesis failure. Catheter Cardiovasc Interv 2016;88:994–1001.
3. Cullen MW, Cabalka AK, Alli OO, et al. Transvenous, antegrade melody valve-in-valve implantation for bioprosthetic mitral and tricuspid valve dysfunction: a case series in children and adults. JACC Cardiovasc Interv 2013;6: 598–605.
4. Kilic A, Saha-Chaudhuri P, Rankin JS, et al. Trends and outcomes of tricuspid valve surgery in north america: an analysis of more than 50,000 patients from the society of thoracic surgeons database. The Ann Thorac Surg 2013;96: 1546–52.
5. Chang B-C, Lim S-H, Yi G, et al. Long-term clinical results of tricuspid valve replacement. The Ann Thorac Surg 2006;81:1317–24.
6. McCarthy PM, Bhudia SK, Rajeswaran J, et al. Tricuspid valve repair: durability and risk factors for failure. The J Thorac Cardiovasc Surg 2004; 127:674–85.
7. Marquis-Gravel G, Bouchard D, Perrault LP, et al. Retrospective cohort analysis of 926 tricuspid valve surgeries: clinical and hemodynamic outcomes with propensity score analysis. Am Heart J 2012; 163:851–8.e1.
8. Vassileva CM, Shabosky J, Boley T, et al. Tricuspid valve surgery: The past 10 years from the Nationwide Inpatient Sample (NIS) database. J Thorac Cardiovasc Surg 2012;143:1043–9.
9. Filsoufi F, Anyanwu AC, Salzberg SP, et al. Long-term outcomes of tricuspid valve replacement in the current era. Ann Thorac Surg 2005;80:845–50.
10. Jones JM, O'Kane H, Gladstone DJ, et al. Repeat heart valve surgery: Risk factors for operative mortality. J Thorac Cardiovasc Surg 2001;122: 913–8.
11. McElhinney DB, Cabalka AK, Aboulhosn JA, et al. Transcatheter tricuspid valve-in-valve implantation for the treatment of dysfunctional surgical bioprosthetic valves: an international, multicenter registry study. Circulation 2016;133:1582–93.
12. McElhinney DB, Aboulhosn JA, Dvir D, et al. Midterm valve-related outcomes after transcatheter tricuspid valve-in-valve or valve-in-ring replacement. J Am Coll Cardiol 2019;73:148–57.
13. Aboulhosn J, Cabalka AK, Levi DS, et al. Transcatheter valve-in-ring implantation for the treatment of residual or recurrent tricuspid valve dysfunction after prior surgical repair. JACC Cardiovasc Interv 2017;10:53–63.
14. Melody™ Transcatheter Pulmonary Valve Instructions for Use. 2019.
15. Anderson JH, McElhinney DB, Aboulhosn J, et al. Management and outcomes of transvenous pacing leads in patients undergoing transcatheter

tricuspid valve replacement. JACC Cardiovasc Interv 2020;13:2012–20.

16. Bapat V. Valve-in-valve apps: why and how they were developed and how to use them. EuroIntervention 2014;10 Suppl. U:U44-51.

17. Hensey M, Alenezi AR, Murdoch DJ, et al. Transcatheter tricuspid valve-in-valve replacement with subsequent bioprosthetic valve fracture to optimize Hemodynamic Function. JACC Cardiovasc Interv 2018;11:2226–7.

18. Mixon TA, Cross DS, Lawrence ME, et al. Temporary coronary guidewire pacing during percutaneous coronary intervention. Catheter Cardiovasc Interv 2004;61:494–500.

Orthotopic Transcatheter Tricuspid Valve Replacement

Adam B. Greenbaum, MD[a], Vasilis C. Babaliaros, MD[a],
Marvin H. Eng, MD[b],*

KEYWORDS
• Tricuspid valve regurgitation • Transcatheter • Tricuspid valve replacement • Percutaneous

KEY POINTS
• Patients with severe tricuspid regurgitation are frequently malnourished, frail, and have hepatic dysfunction–related coagulopathy; this increases their procedural risk and propensity for bleeding postprocedure. • Vigorous anatomic screening with computed tomography is the main driver for determining anatomic eligibility. • Conduction system proximity and ventricular leads from implantable devices are common challenges with transcatheter tricuspid valve replacement (TTVR) cases. Contingencies for the management of heart block should be made ahead of time, as new ventricular leads would compromise a TTVR result. Coronary sinus or leadless pacing is an option for heart block in TTVR. • Patient selection for anticoagulation candidacy should be carefully considered, as nonaccess site bleeding was seen in the early experience of TTVR.

INTRODUCTION

Tricuspid regurgitation (TR), once perceived as a bystander lesion in valvular heart disease, has come into focus as a significant contributor to heart failure and cardiovascular mortality. Based on population studies from Oxford, the prevalence of clinically significant TR is 2.7%[1] and the rate of greater than moderate TR increases with age.[2] The presence of severe TR is associated with a nearly 6-fold odds of mortality.[3] Isolated tricuspid valve surgery has recently been increasing in volume to a rate of ~ 780 cases per year but accompanied by an 8.8% mortality rate.[4] Given the increasing volume of patients with severe TR in the elderly population and the elevated mortality rates of tricuspid valve surgery, percutaneous alternatives have been sought after.

TR is functional approximately 95% of the time, resulting in annular dilation and subsequent leaflet malcoaptation.[5] Over time, the vicious cycle of volume overload, annular dilation, and worsening regurgitation distorts the annulus to the point of severe central malcoaptation. Although registry data indicates the most widely utilized percutaneous tricuspid valve therapy is edge-to-edge repair,[6] this strategy is often inefficacious for patients with very large central malcoaptation. As a result, alternative means to treat TR such as percutaneous annuloplasty or transcatheter tricuspid valve replacement (TTVR) are being investigated.

[a] Structural Heart and Valve Center, Department of Internal Medicine–Cardiology, Emory University, 550 Peachtree St Ne Medical, Office Tower, Fl 6, Atlanta, GA 30308, USA; [b] Division of Cardiology, Structural Heart Program, Banner University Medical Center- Phoenix, University of Arizona, 1111 East McDowell Road, Phoenix, AZ 85006, USA
* Corresponding author.
E-mail address: marvin.eng@bannerhealth.com

Intervent Cardiol Clin 11 (2022) 87–94
https://doi.org/10.1016/j.iccl.2021.09.009
2211-7458/22/© 2021 Elsevier Inc. All rights reserved.

Percutaneous orthotopic TTVR is embarking on its initial stages and iteration of devices. Thus far, the experience has been concentrated in 3 devices: the NaviGate valve (*NaviGate* Cardiac Structures Inc., Lake Forest, CA), the Intrepid valve (Medtronic, Minneapolis, MN), and the Evoque valve (Edwards Lifesciences, Irvine, CA). At this time, the Evoque transcatheter heart valve (THV) is the only device in pivotal clinical trial.

PATIENT EVALUATION AND CASE SELECTION

The insidious nature of the TR renders patients chronically ill and frail. The low-flow state and right-sided edema negatively affects renal function, hepatic function, and bowel wall integrity, causing chronic edema and subsequent malnutrition as a result of protein-losing enteropathy.[7] Therefore, clinicians should be wary of elderly debilitated patients with severe TR as they may have cardiac cirrhosis or have poor overall constitution. Notably in the percutaneous experience with postsurgical failures, older patients or patients with recent hospitalization or acute illness have attenuated survival.[8]

EVOQUE VALVE

The Evoque valve is a large self-expanding prosthesis with bovine pericardial leaflets mounted on nitinol frame (Fig. 1A).[9] The valve uses an anchoring system that uses the annulus, leaflets, and chordal apparatus for fixation. The system is a collection of 9 anchors that grasp the leaflets and chordal apparatus to secure the valve at the tricuspid annulus. The accompanying pericardial skirt is used to minimize paravalvular leak. The delivery system is 28 French (Fr), and there are currently 3 sizes, 44, 48, and 52 mm.

The Evoque delivery system has 3 primary motions: primary flexion to approximate a coaxial plan, a secondary flexion system that moves the delivery system in an oblique direction, and a depth knob to control depth of release (Fig. 1B).

Anatomic considerations and case selection: guiding principles of valve implantation are coaxial alignment and circumferential leaflet capture. Procedural planning for achieving these goals is performed through computed tomography (CT) modeling of device interaction with individualized patient anatomy. Anatomic factors key to planning and eligibility are described later Table 1 and Fig. 2).

Procedural Sequence

The Evoque valve is primarily designed to be deployed via transfemoral venous access and can deploy from either the right or left common femoral vein (Fig. 3). Left access is considered if the CT modeling indicates coaxial alignment or height above the tricuspid annulus is more favorable from the left side. Internal jugular access is being explored as a possible route but it is not considered standard. Systemic anticoagulation should be given to achieve an activated clotting of greater than 300 seconds. Subsequently a deflectable catheter is used to direct a preformed nitinol wire (Safari Extra Small Curl, Boston Scientific, Marlborough, MA) into the right ventricular (RV) apex. After positioning the wire in the ventricular apex, exchange is made for the 28 Fr delivery system. After introducing the valve apparatus across the tricuspid valve, coaxial alignment is optimized. Device depth is then slowly aligned to a position just ventricular to the leaflets, and the anchors are slowly exposed by withdrawing the outer restraining capsule. Use of 2-dimensional (2D) and 3D echocardiography for assessment of leaflet capture is performed circumferentially with multiple iterations during anchor deployment. After the 9 anchors are confirmed to have sufficient leaflet capture, then the valve is slowly expanded to maximum diameter. At times, significant native leaflet retraction at multiple commissures may cause one anchor to fail to capture leaflet. Missing capture of one leaflet is considered acceptable, but 2 consecutive missed anchors could lead to paravalvular regurgitation. Once released, the delivery system is carefully removed and hemostasis achieved either with subcutaneous or previously

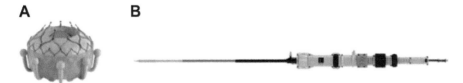

Fig. 1. Evoque transcatheter heart valve and delivery system. (*A*) EVOQUE transcatheter heart valve: self-expanding nitinol frame with bovine pericardial leaflets, intraannular sealing skirt, and ventricular anchors. (*B*) The 28-Fr EVOQUE tricuspid delivery system.

Table 1
Anatomic factors and ramifications for Evoque valve implantation

	Anatomic Factor	Ramifications
Ventricle	Ventricular depth	Insufficient depth may interfere with coaxial alignment (Fig. 2A, dotted white line)
	Subvalvular apparatus density (chordal structures and papillary muscle insertions)	If the valve anchors are released too ventricular, dense subvalvular apparatus may ensnare the anchors and prevent leaflet grasping (see Fig. 2B, white circle)
	Trabecular density and moderator band location	This may bias distal wire position and influence coaxial alignment. The distal wire can become entrapped and prevent freedom of movement of the entire apparatus (see Fig. 2A, white arrow)
Atrial	Inferior vena cava/atrial tortuosity and prominent Eustachian ridge	This may bias the delivery system and hamper maneuvering (see Fig. 2C, black arrow)
	Cardiac-caval angulation	May influence coaxial alignment (see Fig. 2C, white arc)
	Atrial to tricuspid distance	Insufficient height may make leaflet grasping difficult (see Fig. 2C, white bracket)
Leaflets	Leaflet restriction	Severe leaflet restriction with little distance between leaflets and the ventricle may prevent leaflet capture (see Fig. 2A, red circle)
	Leaflet prolapse	Significant segments of the leaflet prolapse may prevent stable THV anchoring
	"Bridge distance"	Distance from the center of the right atrium to the projected location of the delivery system when looking from the short axis perspective of the right ventricle. A longer distance may prevent coaxial alignment (see Fig. 2D, white line)

placed intravascular sutures (Perclose ProGlide, Abbott Vascular, Santa Clara, CA).

Clinical Results

Initial clinical description of the Evoque TTVR describes a single-arm cohort, multicenter study of 25 patients treated on a compassionate basis.[10] All were at high surgical risk with a mean Society of Thoracic Surgery (STS) 30-day predicted mortality of 9.1%, and almost all patients had NYHA functional class III or IV. This early compassionate use cohort was able to achieve 92% technical success, and there were no intraprocedural mortalities. Reduction of TR was less than or equal to 1+ in 92% of patients. At 30 days, mortality was

0%, and there were no valve reinterventions or heart failure hospitalizations. Of note, 2 patients (8%) developed RV afterload mismatch requiring short-term inotropic support. Another 2 patients required permanent pacing postimplant. Three patients suffered major bleeding complications, all related to oral anticoagulation, and none were access related. RV diameter improved on serial imaging at 30 days but RV function as assessed by TAPSE was worse.

The TRISCEND (NCT04221490) trial is a North American multicenter early feasibility study (EFS).[11] The patient population enrolled was elderly (mean age 79 ± years) and high risk for surgery with a mean STS PROM of

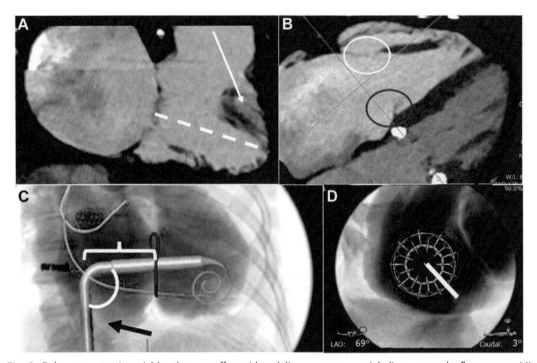

Fig. 2. Relevant anatomic variables that can affect either delivery system coaxial alignment or leaflet capture. (A) Long-axis oblique view of the right atrium and right ventricle displaying ventricular depth (*dotted line*) and apical trabeculae (*white arrow*). (B) Long-axis 4-chambered view depicting papillary muscle-chordal apparatus (*white circle*) and leaflet restriction (*red arrow*). (C) CT modeling of an Evoque delivery catheter showing the height of delivery catheter over the tricuspid annulus (*bracket*) and region of caval-atrial tortuosity (*black arrow*). (D) CT modeling of an Evoque valve with a short-axis perspective. (*Adapted from* [C] Fam, NP et al. JACC: Cardiovascular Interventions 2021;14(3):501-11, permissions granted; and [D] Layoun, H. et al., Current Cardiology Reports 2021;23:114, permissions granted.)

7.7 ± 5.2%. There was a high preponderance of atrial fibrillation (91%) and chronic kidney disease (66%). Nearly all patients had greater than or equal to severe TR (92%). Procedurally, there was 98% rate of device success and 94% rate of procedural success. At 30 days, 2 patients died (3.8%) with one cardiovascular mortality. Severe bleeding occurred in 22.6% of patients. Echocardiography at 30 days found 98% of patients to have nonmild TR. The success of the EFS study has led to the initiation of a pivotal study randomizing device to optimized medical therapy (TRISCEND II, NCT04482062).

NaviGate

There is a limited experience with the GATE system THV (NaviGate Cardiac Structures Inc, Lake Forest, CA) but it is a first-generation valve for TTVR (Fig. 4).[12] The NaviGate valve is a self-expanding nitinol frame with a trileaflet porcine valve. The valve is tapered, and the ventricular outflow is 10 mm larger than the atrial inflow. A combination of 5% to 10% prosthesis

oversizing and 12 atrial winglets and ventricular graspers anchors the valve. It has been deployed via the right internal jugular and transatrial approach with thoracotomy. Currently it uses a 42-Fr sheath and is available in 36, 40, 44, and 52 mm.[13] A report of 30 patients undergoing compassionate use basis demonstrated 87% technical success.[12] Most patients (75%) experienced greater than or equal to 75% reductions in TR. Most implants were transatrial (25/30), and there was a 10% in-hospital mortality. There were a total of 4 technical failures.

LuX-VALVE

LuX-Valve (Jenscare Biotechnology, Ningbo, China) is a novel prosthesis composed of 4 components: (1) trileaflet prosthetic valve with bovine pericardium; (2) self-expanding nitinol valve stent consisting of an atrial disc; (3) 1 interventricular septal anchor "tongue"; and (4) 2 expanded polytetrafluoroethylene-covered graspers (see Fig. 4).[14] The THV is delivered using a 32-Fr catheter through a right thoracotomy and transatrial

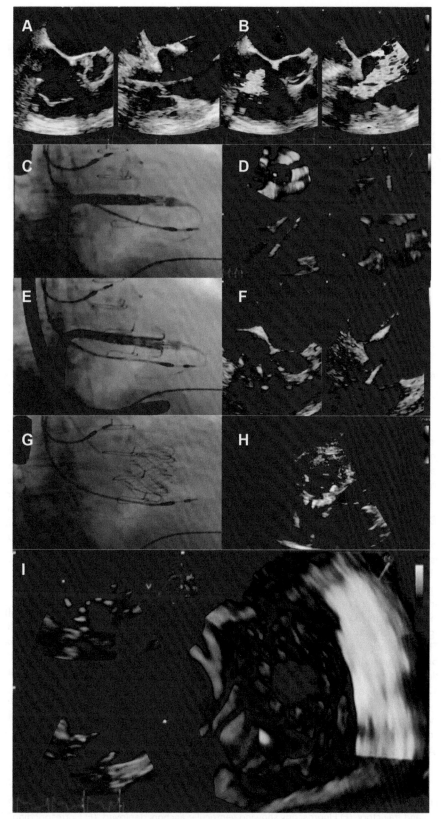

Fig. 3. Deployment sequence of Evoque THV in the tricuspid position. (*A*) Baseline echocardiogram demonstrating lead adherent to posterior tricuspid leaflet. (*B*) Baseline echocardiogram with color Doppler showing massive tricuspid regurgitation (TR). (*C*) Fluoroscopy of initial position of Evoque delivery system across the tricuspid

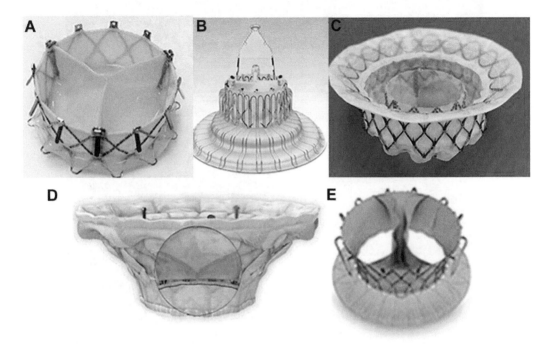

Fig. 4. Burgeoning transcatheter tricuspid valve replacements in early clinical development. (*A*) Gate system; (*B*) LuX-Valve; (*C*) Intrepid; (*D*) Cardiovalve; (*E*) Trisol. ([C] Reproduced with permission of Medtronic, Inc.)

approach using TEE and fluoroscopy. Only a 12-patient report has been documented. In those patients, all had technical success, and there were no procedural mortalities, but one patient died from an acute myocardial infarction postprocedurally.

INTREPID

The Intrepid valve is a trileaflet porcine pericardial prosthesis mounted on a nitinol frame (see Fig. 4).[15] The valve consists of a circular outer fixation frame that comes in 3 sizes (43, 46, or 60 mm) and the inner frame is 27 mm. The valve is fixed to the annulus via oversizing of the self-expanding frame and small cleats that engage leaflets. The atrial portion of the valve is flexible and conforms to the annulus, whereas the ventricular portion is stiffer. Currently it is delivered through a 35-Fr sheath, and for use in the tricuspid position, a transfemoral approach is available currently via surgical cut-down. Early experience has been described, and an early feasibility study is now in progress (NCT04433065).

CARDIOVALVE

Cardiovalve (Boston Medical, Shrewsbury, MA) is a bovine pericardial valve mounted on a nitinol frame that is fixed to the heart by grasping by an atrial flange and a proprietary anchoring and sealing element (see Fig. 4). The valve is delivered through a 28-Fr sheath and available from 45 to 55 mm in 5 mm increments. A US EFS study (NCT04100720) is underway.[13]

TRISOL

Trisol (Trisol Medical, Yokneam, Israel) is a self-expanding conical nitinol frame with a single bovine pericardial dome-shaped leaflet (see Fig. 4). The leaflet is attached in 2 opposite center commissures to create a bileaflet anatomy. It is designed to be deployed via jugular access through a 30-Fr delivery system. First-in-man implantation of the prosthesis was reported to be successful in a patient with high surgical risk.[16]

annulus. (*D*) Corresponding 3-dimensional (3D) transesophageal echocardiographic (TEE) imaging of delivery system position and trajectory. (*E*) Fluoroscopy showing ventricular anchors deployed. (*F*) Corresponding 3D TEE imaging of tricuspid leaflet capture. (*G*) Fluoroscopy after atrial expansion and valve release. (*H*) Transthoracic echocardiography at follow-up showing trace TR. (*I*) 3D TEE imaging showing pacemaker lead in posteroseptal commissure.[10]

OTHER CONSIDERATIONS FOR TRICUSPID VALVE REPLACEMENT

Postprocedure Anticoagulation

There is no consensus on preferred anticoagulation agents or duration of thrombosis prophylaxis. The TRISCEND II mandates up to 6 months of anticoagulation with warfarin (international normalized ratio: INR 2–3) and aspirin 81 mg daily. Prior experience with an off-label balloon expandable valve use showed that among 302 patients, 50% of them were discharged with oral anticoagulation, and there was a cumulative incidence of thrombosis of 0.033 (0.015—0.061 at 3 years.[8] A higher post-TTVR gradient was associated with an increased risk for thrombosis (heart rate 1.38 per mmHg). Given the relative high rate of nonaccess site bleeding observed in the TRISCEND EFS, patient selection for bleeding risk will be important.[11]

CONDUCTION ABNORMALITIES AND MANAGEMENT OF TRANSVENOUS ELECTRICAL LEADS

Proximity of the atrioventricular node and His-Purkinje system makes patients vulnerable to conduction system injury with placement of devices in the tricuspid annulus. Placing a THV in the tricuspid position will exclude patients from usual ventricular lead placement, and special contingencies will need to be planned should heart block occur. Of note, 34% of the TRISCEND EFS study had pacemakers or intracardiac defibrillators (ICD), indicating that ventricular lead placement is common among the severe TR population.[11] Patients that are pacer dependent or who had ICDs implanted for secondary sudden prevention will require forethought should the ventricular leads be compromised by THV implantation. Leadless pacemakers or coronary sinus lead placement have been widely used in the event of heart block or compromised pacing leads, and a treatment plan should be clearly delineated before proceeding.

RIGHT HEART FAILURE

Patients with severe TR may have associated RV dilation and systolic dysfunction. Correcting TR may further unmask RV dysfunction and possibly even cause hemodynamic compromise. As seen already, 2 patients in the early EVOQUE experience required inotropes for ventricular support postimplantation.[10] Patient selection and understanding which patients may not be suitable for valve implantation will need to be further explored in upcoming studies. Involvement of advanced heart failure experts in the postprocedure management should be considered for the patients with preexisting systolic dysfunction and torrential TR.

SUMMARY

Patients with severe TR are high risk for surgery, and tricuspid surgery is associated with high mortality, making transcatheter therapies a high priority for patients with TR. The functional nature of most TR leads to large coaptation gaps, and this favors valve replacement over repair; therefore, we should expect TTVR to have a significant impact. Future studies will need to determine patient selection, prosthesis efficacy, duration of thromboprophylaxis, and prothesis durability. With percutaneous tricuspid replacement, correction of valvular regurgitation will be feasible even in the most challenging patient anatomies.

CLINICS CARE POINTS

- Severe tricuspid regurgitation is a major contributor to cardiovascular mortality and morbidity.

- The insidious nature of tricuspid regurgitation renders patients frail, malnourished and causes liver dysfunction.

- Orthotopic valve replacement heavily relies on multimodality imaging to determine anatomic suitability.

DISCLOSURES

Marvin H. Eng, MD is a clinical proctor for Edwards Lifesciences and Medtronic. V. Babaliaros is a consultant for Edwards Lifesciences. A.B. Greenbaum is a consultant to Edwards Lifesciences, Medtronic, and Abbott.

REFERENCES

1. d'Arcy JL, Coffey S, Loudon MA, et al. Large-scale community echocardiographic screening reveals a major burden of undiagnosed valvular heart disease in older people: the OxVALVE Population Cohort Study. Eur Heart J 2016;37:3515–22.

2. Topilsky Y, Maltais S, Medina Inojosa J, et al. Burden of tricuspid regurgitation in patients diagnosed in the community setting. JACC Cardiovasc Imaging 2019;12:433–42.

3. Nath J, Foster E, Heidenreich PA. Impact of tricuspid regurgitation on long-term survival. J Am Coll Cardiol 2004;43:405–9.

4. Zack CJ, Fender EA, Chandrashekar P, et al. National trends and outcomes in isolated tricuspid valve surgery. J Am Coll Cardiol 2017;70:2953–60.

5. Prihadi EA, van der Bijl P, Gursoy E, et al. Development of significant tricuspid regurgitation over time and prognostic implications: new insights into natural history. Eur Heart J 2018;39:3574–81.

6. Taramasso M, Alessandrini H, Latib A, et al. Outcomes after current transcatheter tricuspid valve intervention: mid-term results from the international trivalve registry. JACC Cardiovasc Interv 2019;12:155–65.

7. Besler C, Orban M, Rommel K-P, et al. Predictors of procedural and clinical outcomes in patients with symptomatic tricuspid regurgitation undergoing transcatheter edge-to-edge repair. JACC Cardiovasc Interv 2018;11:1119–28.

8. McElhinney DB, Aboulhosn JA, Dvir D, et al. Mid-term valve-related outcomes after transcatheter tricuspid valve-in-valve or valve-in-ring replacement. J Am Coll Cardiol 2019;73:148–57.

9. Fam NP, Ong G, Deva DP, et al. Transfemoral transcatheter tricuspid valve replacement. JACC Cardiovasc Interv 2020;13:e93–4.

10. Fam NP, von Bardeleben RS, Hensey M, et al. Transfemoral transcatheter tricuspid valve replacement with the evoque system: a multicenter, observational, first-in-human experience. JACC Cardiovasc Interv 2021;14:501–11.

11. Kodali Susheel K. Transfemoral tricuspid valve replacement in patients with tricuspid regurgitation: 30-day results of the triscend study. Am Coll Cardiol 2021.

12. Hahn RT, Kodali S, Fam N, et al. Early multinational experience of transcatheter tricuspid valve replacement for treating severe tricuspid regurgitation. JACC Cardiovasc Interv 2020;13:2482–93.

13. Goldberg YH, Ho E, Chau M, et al. Update on transcatheter tricuspid valve replacement therapies. Front Cardiovasc Med 2021;8:619558.

14. Lu F-L, Ma Y, An Z, et al. First-in-man experience of transcatheter tricuspid valve replacement with lux-valve in high-risk tricuspid regurgitation patients. JACC Cardiovasc Interv 2020;13:1614–6.

15. Bapat V. The INTREPID valve for severe tricuspid regurgitation: case experience. Washington, DC: CRT 2020; 2020.

16. Vaturi M, Vaknin-Assa H, Shapira Y, et al. First-in-human percutaneous transcatheter tricuspid valve replacement with a novel valve. JACC Case Rep 2021;3:1281–6.

Caval Valve Implantation

Alexander Lauten, MD[a,b,*], Henryk Dreger, MD[c], Michael Laule, MD[c],
Karl Stangl, MD[c], Hans R. Figulla, MD[d], Marvin H. Eng, MD[e]

KEYWORDS

- Caval valve implantation • Tricuspid valve regurgitation • Tricuspid valve insufficiency
- Right heart failure • Functional tricuspid regurgitation

KEY POINTS

- Frailty and significant dilation of the tricuspid annulus frequently renders patients ineligible for surgical therapy or percutaneous repair of the tricuspid valve, respectively.
- Heterotopic valve implantation was devised as a creative means to prevent the pressurization of the venous system from tricuspid valve regurgitation.
- Owing to the exceeding frailty of patients, there is high early mortality related to chronic illness and comorbidities.

INTRODUCTION

Recently, transcatheter therapy has expanded the treatment options for patients with heart valve disease. Interventional therapy for aortic, mitral, and pulmonic valve disease is well established; however, catheter-based approaches to tricuspid regurgitation (TR) are still in early stages of development.[1–4] Traditionally, TR assumed a lower priority than other valve disease, also driven by less commercial interest in such developments in the past. Nevertheless, the prevalence and the functional impact of moderate to severe TR are high, and this disease is currently vastly under-treated.[5] With increasing severity of TR, 1-year mortality increases, reaching greater than 36% in those with severe TR.[6] Furthermore, the increasing number of patients at advanced age and high-risk profile undergoing successful treatment of left heart disease may contribute further to the growing need for effective interventional approaches of TR, because many of these potentially develop right heart disease at a later stage.[7,8]

For some of the interventional concepts to TR—including the edge-to-edge-repair, transcatheter annuloplasty, the tricuspid spacer, and caval valves—procedural feasibility and favorable early clinical outcome have been demonstrated in small compassionate case series.[9–12] However, there is still a lack of evidence and data from randomized trials to demonstrate the functional impact of these treatment approaches. Furthermore, we need a better understanding of clinical and anatomic selection criteria for these approaches as well as a uniform definition of achievable end points, which may differ depending on the subgroup of patients and treatment approaches.[13–15] This article reviews the pathophysiological background and current evidence for caval valve implantation and examines the potential role of this approach for the treatment of severe TR.

Transcatheter Treatment of TR: Orthotopic Versus Heterotopic Replacement

Although percutaneous repair concepts are conceptually attractive because they restore native tricuspid valve function, it remains

This article was previously published in *Interventional Cardiology Clinics*, Volume 7, Number 1, Pages 57-63.
[a] Helios Klinikum Erfurt GmbH, Erfurt, Thuringia, Germany; [b] Department of Cardiology, Helios Clinic Erfurt, Nordhauser StraBe 74, Erfurt 99089, Germany; [c] Charité–University Hospital Berlin, Berlin, Germany; [d] University Heart Center Jena, Germany; [e] Banner University Medical Center, 1111 East McDowell Road, Phoenix, AZ 85006, USA
* Corresponding author. Department of Cardiology, Helios Clinic Erfurt, Nordhauser StraBe 74, Erfurt 99089, Germany.
E-mail address: alelau2015@gmx.de

arguable to what extent repair concepts can be implemented on the tricuspid valve with durable long-term results. Repair does not encompass all tricuspid pathology; especially patients with large coaptation gaps are not suitable repair candidates due to lack of efficacy. Because of the above-mentioned unmet need for an effective treatment, transcatheter valve implantation may be an alternative and easier-to-achieve treatment option.

From the interventional perspective, there are 2 basic principles depending on the site of valve implantation—an *orthotopic* versus a *heterotopic, caval* valve implantation. For *orthotopic* valve replacement, the prosthetic valve is implanted in anatomically correct position in the TV annulus, thus restoring the functional separation of the right ventricle (RV) and right atrium (RA). Repair and heterotopic replacement tends to only partially correct TR thus reducing the hemodynamic burden of acute complete correction to the RV, whereas the orthotopic approach will most likely lead to complete correction of ventricular regurgitation. It remains arguable whether this is necessary to achieve clinical improvement or is hemodynamically desirable in patients with RV dysfunction.

Furthermore, the orthotopic approach is associated with particular challenges in patients with severe and long-standing TR. At present, only investigational devices are available; they are in early stages of clinical development and only one is in a prospective pivotal study (TRISCEND II NCT04482062). Compared with the aortic annulus, the TV annulus offers a greater variability and less resistance for device fixation because of its larger diameter and lower proportion of fibrous tissue. Size and flexibility of the TV and the surrounding myocardium hamper positioning and long-term fixation of transcatheter devices, and there are no adjacent structures to facilitate implantation of such devices. Annulus dilatation may reach greater than 70 mm in functional TR and is associated with the loss of anatomic landmarks between RV and RA. A device intended for orthotopic TV replacement would require unique solutions for stent and catheter design as well as tissue valve engineering (eg, a 70-mm tissue valve would require a leaflet height of >40 mm to avoid prolapsing into the RA). In 2005, Boudjemline and colleagues[16] experimentally investigated this approach by implanting a double-disk nitinol stent with a semilunar valve into the TV annulus. Although in this study technical feasibility was demonstrated to some degree in healthy sheep, several difficulties relating to sufficient fixation

of the self-expanding valve in the highly dynamic tricuspid annulus were observed.[16]

Heterotopic, caval valve implantation is an obviously attractive alternative. Compared with the *orthotopic* approach, the heterotopic procedure benefits from the advantage of a straightforward implantation technique owing to the distance to vulnerable cardiac structures. The introduction of foreign material in the RV inflow tract is avoided, permitting a potentially lower risk of injury to ventricular structures and making this an attractive approach to the interventional cardiologist. Devices do not interfere with any preexisting transtricuspid pacemaker or defibrillator leads, which might represent a limitation for orthotopic procedures on the tricuspid valve.

The CAVI Approach: from Preclinical Proof of Concept to First Human Application

The CAVI concept was first investigated in an experimental study in animals demonstrating function and hemodynamic effects of the caval valves. After creation of acute TR in sheep, self-expanding valves were implanted in the inferior vena cava (IVC) and superior vena cava (SVC) using a transjugular approach (Fig. 1A). In this study, the onset of TR resulted in a significant reduction of cardiac output and a ventricular wave in the IVC. After implantation of the IVC and SVC valves, cardiac output and systolic backflow in the caval veins recovered to baseline value.[15,17] Chronic animal data demonstrated device function for a period of up to 6 months after implantation (Fig. 1B, C).[18]

After demonstration of feasibility, CAVI was first applied for compassionate treatment in a human patient in 2010.[13] In this patient with severe functional TR after multiple preceding open-heart procedures, a self-expanding valve was implanted into the IVC at the cavoatrial junction to reduce regurgitant backflow. In this experience, excellent valve function was observed after deployment resulting in a marked reduction of caval pressure and an abolition of backflow to the IVC (Fig. 1D, E). The patient was discharged home and experienced an improvement of physical capacity and symptoms of right heart failure within the 3-month follow-up period.[19] The first series of patients treated with caval implantation of the Edwards Sapien XT (Edwards Lifesciences, Irvine, CA, USA) valve was published by Laule and colleagues[20] in 2013, reporting the experience with IVC implantation of balloon-expandable valves (BEVs) in 3 patients with severe functional TR (Fig. 1F, G).

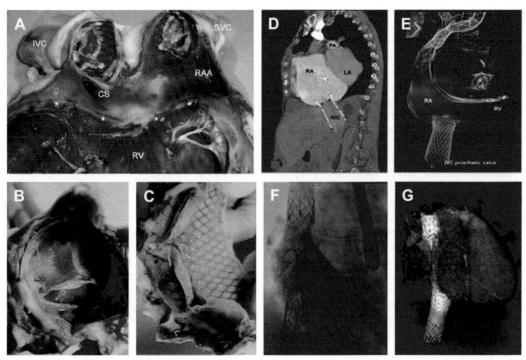

Fig. 1. From preclinical proof of concept to first human application. (A–C) Preclinical proof of concept was demonstrated in a sheep model of acute severe TR. The onset of TR resulted in a significant reduction of cardiac output and a ventricular wave in the inferior vena cava. After implantation of the IVC and SVC valves, cardiac output and systolic backflow in the caval veins recovered to baseline. Chronic animal data demonstrated device function for a period of up to 6 months after implantation. First-in-man demonstrated feasibility using custom-made devices for IVC only (D, E) and Edwards Sapien XT valves for bicaval implantation (F, G). LA, left atrium.

Clinical Evidence

With our growing understanding of TR and its natural history it becomes more and more obvious that this patient population is actually a heterogeneous cohort presenting for treatment in different stages of a continuous disease process. It is yet unclear which interventional approach will result in functional and clinical success and in which subtype of patient population. The various interventional approaches that are under development today, including edge-to-edge-repair, annuloplasty, and the caval approach, potentially focus at different subgroups of patients with TR and may also require different measures of outcome depending on the disease stage.[11,12,21,22]

A recent observational study summarizes the current experience with CAVI in a multicenter series of 25 patients.[23] The study demonstrates that treatment of severe TR with the CAVI technique is feasible, safe, and hemodynamically effective. Successful implantation of either self-expandable valve or BEVs resulted in the resolution of caval backflow in all patients, and treatment further translated into New York Heart

Association class improvement. However, with a mean STS score of 14.0 ± 12.7, the study included a high proportion of excessive risk patients and therefore showed a 12% and 24% 30-day and in-hospital mortalities, respectively. Most patients underwent single valve implantation (76%), and the remainder had bicaval implantation with either balloon-expandable (Sapien XT) or self-expanding valves (TricValve, P&F, Vienna, Austria). Procedural success was 92% with no procedural deaths. Two valve migrations with conversions to open heart surgery occurred, one case immediately after implantation and another postdischarge. Hemodynamically, the most significant improvements were observed in IVC and RA pressure. Echocardiographic markers of RV function did not change.

Follow-up to the initial clinical experience is an investigator-initiated, prospective, randomized trial named TRICAVAL (Treatment of Severe Secondary Tricuspid Regurgitation in Patients with Advance Heart Failure with Caval Vein Implantation of the Edwards Sapien XT Valve; NCT02387697).[24] The primary end point was exercise capacity as measured by treadmill spiroergometry at 3 months, and the study randomized 28 patients 1:1 to device:medical therapy. The study was stopped early due to delayed major complications related to stent (2) and valve (2) migration. For the surviving patients, there was no difference in exercise capacity or symptoms over long-term follow-up. The CAVI group had 21% and 57% in-hospital and 12-month mortalities, respectively, whereas the medical group had 29% mortality.

Documentation of other early experience includes a 24-patient North American series of IVC-only implantations with the Edwards Sapien 3 (Edwards Lifesciences, Irvine, CA, USA) valve.[25] In this series, in-hospital and 30-day follow-up were 20.8% and 25%, respectively. Survival at the median follow-up of 332 days was 58.3%, in line with the notion that patients with decompensated severe TR are frail and have poor life expectancy. Other smaller series have been published suggesting that hemodynamic indices could be improved, but a longitudinal study demonstrating durable efficacy of heterotopic implantation has yet to be published.[26,27] Forthcoming studies in newer valves such as the TricValve and Tricento (New Valve Technology, Muri, Switzerland) may be forthcoming and may provide fresh insight into the potential salutary impact of heterotopic valve implantation.[28,29]

Anatomic and Hemodynamic Patient Selection

Patients with significant TR may remain asymptomatic for many years. However, because TR frequently develops with the progression of left heart or pulmonary disease, the underlying disorder rather than the tricuspid valve lesion tends to dominate the clinical picture. Increased RA pressure is transmitted to the central and hepatic veins leading to hepatosplenomegaly and ascites, which are present in 90% of patients with severe TR.[5,30] In the advanced disease stage, TR and associated right heart failure are associated with a wide range of hemodynamic and anatomic alterations, including massive dilatation and elongation of the IVC and SVC. Because RV stroke volume is partially expelled backward into the venous system, there is a resulting decrease in cardiac output and RV afterload. This decrease in RV afterload in the presence of TR may initially actually mask a decreased RV contractility. However, increasing volume overload contributes to further RV and tricuspid annulus dilatation leading to a worsening of TR. As RV preload increases, the RV further loses its contractility and eventually fails.

Pulsatile blood flow and systolic flow reversal in the caval veins are prerequisites for the proper function of the caval valves; hemodynamic proof of regurgitation is required before heterotopic implantation. Therefore, caval valve implantation is likely to be effective only in patients with preserved RV function. The prognostic significance of preserved RV function is already known to affect the outcome after tricuspid valve surgery, and will probably to a certain degree also impact outcome after any interventional tricuspid valve procedure.

When screening patients for CAVI, understanding the changes of venous anatomy associated with TR is of importance. In severe TR, the IVC dilates in the upper abdominal section below the diaphragm, frequently reaching diameters ~45 mm below the inflow of the hepatic veins. Owing to the constraining outer fibrous structure of the crossing through the diaphragm, the uppermost IVC section hardly dilates. Thus, this section serves as the preferred landing zone for secure valve implantation.

In contrast, the inflow section of the SVC into the RA tends to massively dilate, particularly the venous segment below the level of the right pulmonary artery; this leads to atrialization of the distal venous segment and results in a tapered anatomy, which makes sufficient valve fixation difficult. A wide variability of venous diameters can be found in patients with severe TR, requiring dedicated devices that provide sufficient anchoring in most anatomies (Fig. 2).

Under the condition of severe TR, the anatomic diameter of the SVC and IVC frequently exceeds the suitable range for implantation of current commercially available devices. Regarding the Edwards Sapien XT or Sapien 3 valve, this has been partially compensated for by prestenting the caval veins before valve deployment for downsizing and improved valve anchoring.

Current CAVI experience includes the implantation of the balloon-expandable Edwards Sapien XT or Sapien 3 and the self-expandable TricValve. Neither device is yet approved for venous implantation; all implantations have been performed under compassionate clinical use or within clinical study protocols.

Anatomic screening and decision for single versus bicaval implantation depended on the available devices. For implantation of BEVs, an IVC diameter at the diaphragmatic intersection and an SVC diameter at the atrial inflow of 30 mm or less are suitable for valve implantation. Furthermore, a tapered anatomy or severe venous elongation of the SVC at the designated

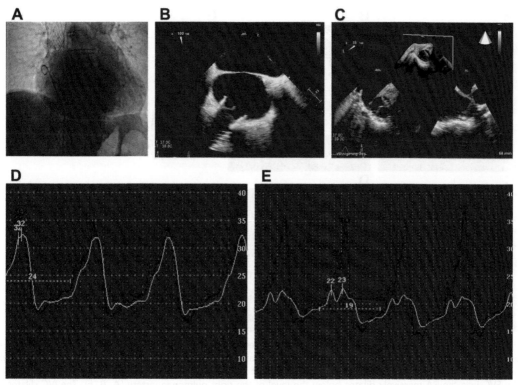

Fig. 2. BiCaval valve implantation using the self-expandable TricValve. (*A–C*) Fluoroscopy and transesophageal echo demonstrate the position and function of the dedicated devices in the SVC and IVC. Angiography (*A*) and invasive pressure tracings (*D, E*) confirm the complete resolution of caval backflow and a marked reduction of the v-wave and mean pressure in the IVC.

landing zone was considered as unsuitable. Anatomic exclusion criteria for TricValve implantation include an IVC diameter at the diaphragmatic intersection and an SVC diameter at the SVC right pulmonary artery crossing of greater than 35 mm (Fig. 3).

How to Perform Caval Valve Implantation

Owing to the commercial availability of the Edwards Sapien XT and Sapien 3 valves for treatment of aortic stenosis (29 mm Edwards Sapien XT or Sapien 3,), there is a growing experience in the off-label use of these devices for CAVI. Although the use of BEV has been commonly limited to the IVC, in selected cases the long segment of the SVC facilitates BEV implantation using the same implant technique. The anatomy of the cavoatrial junction of the IVC (particularly the large diameter, the inflow of hepatic veins, and the compliance of the venous wall) precludes direct implantation of a BEV and requires the preparation of a landing zone by implanting a self-expandable stent to facilitate valve fixation. Thus, a self-expandable stent tailored to IVC diameter (eg, 30 × 80 mm) is implanted in the IVC at

the level of the diaphragm and protruding approximately 5 mm into the RA. The 29-mm BEV mounted on the delivery system is then deployed inside the stent with the lower part just superior to the confluence of the first hepatic vein.

The TricValve is designed as a set of 2 self-expandable valves dedicated for SVC and IVC implantation in the low-pressure circulation. The SVC valve is a belly-shaped tapered device for anchoring in dilated, tapered SVC configuration. The IVC valve is deployed at the level of the diaphragm and protruding into the RA. Both devices are made of bovine pericardium, and the inner part of the atrial stent portion is lined with a PTFE skirt. Both valves are loaded into 27F catheters for sheathless implantation. Before SVC valve implantation, a catheter is placed distally in the right pulmonary artery as marker of the IVC-rPA crossing. The SVC valve is then deployed with the landing zone of the enlarged midportion of the stent above the rPA. The IVC valve is deployed with the upper, skirt-lined segment of the stent protruding into the RA and the device fully deployed and anchored in the SVC.

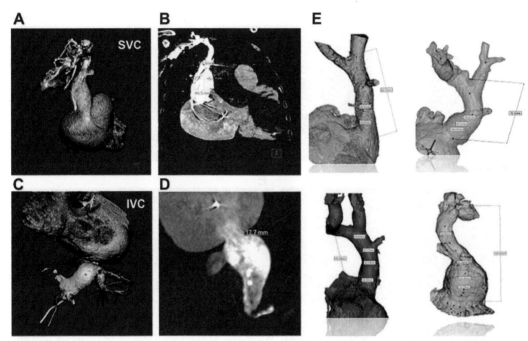

Fig. 3. Changes of venous anatomy associated with severe tricuspid regurgitation. Long-standing severe TR is associated with dilatation and elongation of the inferior and superior venae cavae with the diameter frequently exceeding the suitable range for implantation of current commercially available devices. The inflow section of the SVC into the RA massively dilates below the level of the right pulmonary artery (A, B, E). The IVC dilates in the upper abdominal section below the diaphragm but remains constrained by the diaphragm (C, D).

Potential Limitations

Although caval valve implantation is a rather simple procedure, this approach has important limitations currently restricting its use to nonsurgical patients with symptomatic TR in advanced-stage heart disease.

Nevertheless, limitations apply as well to heterotopic procedures. From a hemodynamic perspective, CAVI does not address TR itself but the regurgitation of blood into the caval veins. As this condition is present only in a subgroup of patients with severe, often long-standing TR and RV enlargement, hemodynamic proof of caval regurgitation is essential before valve implantation. Also it is yet unclear whether this subpopulation benefits from an interventional procedure. The persistence of RA volume overload and the ventricularization of the RA are potential limitations of the procedure; its long-term impact on RA and ventricular function is currently unknown. Although follow-up data in small patient series demonstrate no further RA enlargement up to 12 months after implantation, further evaluation with long term follow-up is required.[31]

Furthermore, caval valve implantation addresses the regurgitation of blood in the caval veins only, a condition not found in every patient with severe TR. In this condition, the RA functions as a compliant reservoir by retaining part of the regurgitant volume and thus limiting systolic flow reversal in the caval veins. Therefore, only patients with proven systolic flow reversal in the caval veins and preserved RV function potentially benefit from this treatment. Furthermore, symptoms of right heart congestion are caused by elevation of mean IVC pressure, which may be slightly reduced after caval valve implantation. Current experience shows, however, that due to RV dysfunction and elevation of mean RA pressure, vena cava pressure is not normalized after caval valve implantation but still remains elevated, which also limits the hemodynamic and functional benefit of the procedure.

SUMMARY

For a large number of patients with functional TR in an advanced stage of multivalvular heart disease, a readily available transcatheter approach could offer an effective treatment option. Their number is likely to increase in the future due to the demographic development and the widespread application of interventional therapies for left heart valve disease. In carefully selected patients, caval valve implantation is a technically straightforward interventional technique and has been applied successfully for compassionate treatment in human patients. Hemodynamic improvement has been consistently observed; however, the clinical benefit of the procedure still requires further evaluation and important hemodynamic limitations apply. As for any other treatment concept of TR, it remains to be determined which patients benefit most from this approach and which outcome measures are most suitable.

DISCLOSURE

A. Lauten: Consultant to P&F TricValve, receives research support from Edwards Lifesciences. H. Dreger reports grants from Edwards Lifesciences. H.R. Figulla is a consultant to P&F TricValve and the founder of JenaValve; K. Stangle reports grants from Edwards Lifesciences and speaker and proctor fees from Abbott, Edwards Lifesciences and Medtronic. M. Laule reports grants from Edwards Lifesciences and Berlin Institute of Health and speaker and proctor fees from Abbott, Edwards Lifesciences, and Medtronic. Marvin H. Eng is a proctor for Edwards Lifesciences and Medtronic.

REFERENCES

1. Leon MB, Smith CR, Mack MJ, et al. Transcatheter or Surgical Aortic-Valve Replacement in Intermediate-Risk Patients. N Engl J Med 2016; 374:1609–20.

2. Figulla HR, Webb JG, Lauten A, et al. The transcatheter valve technology pipeline for treatment of adult valvular heart disease. Eur Heart J 2016; 37:2226–39.

3. Lauten A, Figulla HR, Mollmann H, et al. TAVI for low-flow, low-gradient severe aortic stenosis with preserved or reduced ejection fraction: a subgroup analysis from the German Aortic Valve Registry (GARY). EuroIntervention 2014;10:850–9.

4. Latib A, Mangieri A, Agricola E, et al. Percutaneous bicuspidalization of the tricuspid valve using the MitraClip system. Int J Cardiovasc Imaging 2017; 33:227–8.

5. Stuge O, Liddicoat J. Emerging opportunities for cardiac surgeons within structural heart disease. J Thorac Cardiovasc Surg 2006;132:1258–61.

6. Nath J, Foster E, Heidenreich PA. Impact of tricuspid regurgitation on long-term survival. J Am Coll Cardiol 2004;43:405–9.

7. Rogers JH, Bolling SF. The tricuspid valve: current perspective and evolving management of tricuspid regurgitation. Circulation 2009;119:2718–25.

8. Selle A, Figulla HR, Ferrari M, et al. Impact of rapid ventricular pacing during TAVI on microvascular tissue perfusion. Clin Res Cardiol 2014;103:902–11.

9. Rodes-Cabau J, Hahn RT, Latib A, et al. Transcatheter Therapies for Treating Tricuspid Regurgitation. J Am Coll Cardiol 2016;67:1829–45.

10. Campelo-Parada F, Perlman G, Philippon F, et al. First-in-Man Experience of a Novel Transcatheter Repair System for Treating Severe Tricuspid Regurgitation. J Am Coll Cardiol 2015;66:2475–83.

11. Schofer J, Bijuklic K, Tiburtius C, et al. First-in-human transcatheter tricuspid valve repair in a patient with severely regurgitant tricuspid valve. J Am Coll Cardiol 2015;65:1190–5.

12. Nickenig G, Kowalski M, Hausleiter J, et al. Transcatheter Treatment of Severe Tricuspid Regurgitation With the Edge-to-Edge MitraClip Technique. Circulation 2017;135:1802–14.

13. Lauten A, Ferrari M, Hekmat K, et al. Heterotopic transcatheter tricuspid valve implantation: first-in-man application of a novel approach to tricuspid regurgitation. Eur Heart J 2011;32:1207–13.

14. Mangieri A, Montalto C, Pagnesi M, et al. Mechanism and Implications of the Tricuspid Regurgitation: From the Pathophysiology to the Current and Future Therapeutic Options. Circ Cardiovasc Interv 2017;10(7):e005043.

15. Lauten A, Figulla HR, Willich C, et al. Percutaneous caval stent valve implantation: investigation of an interventional approach for treatment of tricuspid regurgitation. Eur Heart J 2010;31:1274–81.

16. Boudjemline Y, Agnoletti G, Bonnet D, et al. Steps toward the percutaneous replacement of atrioventricular valves an experimental study. J Am Coll Cardiol 2005;46:360–5.

17. Lauten A, Figulla HR, Willich C, et al. Heterotopic valve replacement as an interventional approach to tricuspid regurgitation. J Am Coll Cardiol 2010; 55:499–500.

18. Lauten A, Laube A, Schubert H, et al. Transcatheter treatment of tricuspid regurgitation by caval valve implantation–experimental evaluation of decellularized tissue valves in central venous position. Catheter Cardiovasc Interv 2015;85:150–60.

19. Lauten A, Hamadanchi A, Doenst T, et al. Caval valve implantation for treatment of tricuspid regurgitation: post-mortem evaluation after mid-term follow-up. Eur Heart J 2014;35:1651.

20. Laule M, Stangl V, Sanad W, et al. Percutaneous transfemoral management of severe secondary tricuspid regurgitation with Edwards Sapien XT bioprosthesis: first-in-man experience. J Am Coll Cardiol 2013;61:1929–31.

21. Rosser BA, Taramasso M, Maisano F. Transcatheter interventions for tricuspid regurgitation: TriCinch (4Tech). EuroIntervention 2016;12:Y110–2.

22. Latib A, Agricola E, Pozzoli A, et al. First-in-Man Implantation of a Tricuspid Annular Remodeling Device for Functional Tricuspid Regurgitation. JACC Cardiovasc Interv 2015;8:e211–4.

23. Lauten A, Figulla HR, Unbehaun A, et al. Interventional Treatment of Severe Tricuspid Regurgitation: Early Clinical Experience in a Multicenter, Observational, First-in-Man Study. Circ Cardiovasc Interv 2018;11:e006061.

24. Henryk D, Isabel M, Bernd H, et al. Treatment of Severe TRIcuspid Regurgitation in Patients with Advanced Heart Failure with CAval Vein Implantation of the Edwards Sapien XT VALve (TRICAVAL): a randomised controlled trial. EuroIntervention 2020;15:1506–13.

25. O'Neill B, Negrotto S, Yu D, et al. Cava Valve Implantation for Tricuspid Regurgitation: Insights From the United States Caval Valve Registry. J Invasive Cardiol 2020;32:470–5.

26. Aalaei-Andabili SH, Bavry AA, Choi C, et al. Percutaneous Inferior Vena Cava Valve Implantation May Improve Tricuspid Valve Regurgitation and Cardiac Output: Lessons Learned. Innovations 2020;15:577–80.

27. Sharkey A, Munoz Acuna R, Belani K, et al. Heterotopic caval valve implantation for the management of severe tricuspid regurgitation: a case series. Eur Heart J Case Rep 2020;5:ytaa428.

28. Stefan T, Bart De B, Miriam B, et al. First-in-man implantation of the Tricento transcatheter heart valve for the treatment of severe tricuspid regurgitation. EuroIntervention 2018;14:758–61.

29. Wilbring M, Tomala J, Ulbrich S, et al. Recurrence of Right Heart Failure After Heterotopic Tricuspid Intervention: A Conceptual Misunderstanding? JACC Cardiovasc Interv 2020;13:e95–6.

30. Singh JP, Evans JC, Levy D, et al. Prevalence and clinical determinants of mitral, tricuspid, and aortic regurgitation (the Framingham Heart Study). Am J Cardiol 1999;83:897–902.

31. Lauten A, Figulla HR, Sinning JM, Unbehaun A, Fam N, Schofer J, Doenst T, Hausleiter J, Franz M, Jung C, Dreger H, Leistner D, Stundl A, Landmesser U, Falk V, Stangl K and Laule M. Transcatheter Treatment of Severe Tricuspid Regurgitation using Caval Valve Implantation (CAVI). submitted for publication.

The Role of Intracardiac Echocardiography in Percutaneous Tricuspid Intervention: A New ICE Age

Daniel Hagemeyer, MD[a], Faeez M. Ali, MD[a,b],
Geraldine Ong, MD, MSc[a], Neil P. Fam, MD, MSc[a,*]

KEYWORDS

• Intracardiac echocardiography • Tricuspid valve interventions • Tricuspid regurgitation
• Transcatheter tricuspid valve repair • Intraprocedural guidance • Structural cardiac disorders
• ICE

KEY POINTS

• In percutaneous tricuspid valve intervention, it can be challenging to visualize the anatomy of the valve adequately with transesophageal echocardiography (TEE) due to anatomic limitations, and occasionally TEE is contraindicated.
• Although intracardiac echocardiography (ICE) can improve patients safety by avoiding general anesthesia, its use increases costs and has an operator learning curve.
• In the future, 4D ICE with wider acquisition volumes and real-time multiplanar reconstruction has the potential to replace TEE for procedural guidance.

INTRODUCTION

The burden of tricuspid regurgitation (TR) is high in an aging population.[1] The 1-year survival rate for patients with severe TR is poor (64%).[2] For many years, medical therapy was considered the gold standard. In recent years, evidence has emerged linking right ventricular (RV) volume overload due to chronic TR to irreversible RV myocardial damage and increased mortality.[2–4] Owing to the often silent yet progressive nature of TR, patients often present late, with severe signs of right-sided heart failure, significant tricuspid annular dilatation, and leaflet tethering. For many of these patients, surgery is associated with high perioperative mortality.[5] Therefore, different transcatheter treatment strategies have been developed, and currently, 3 approaches are investigated: edge-to-edge repair, annuloplasty, and valve replacement. Edge-to-edge repair has shown to be feasible for tricuspid repair with both the TriClip (Abbott Vascular, Santa Clara, CA, USA) and the PASCAL device (Edwards Lifesciences, Irvine, CA, USA).[6,7] Long-term outcome data are still missing, but existing data have shown significant clinical improvement after 1 year for transcatheter tricuspid edge-to-edge repair.[8,9] For patients with predominant annular dilatation, reconstruction of the tricuspid annulus with a transfemoral direct annuloplasty with the Cardioband device (Edwards Lifesciences) has shown promising results after 6-month follow-up.[10,11] In contrast to repair devices, transcatheter tricuspid valve replacement using the EVO-QUE device (Edwards Lifesciences) definitively abolishes TR and is now moving into pivotal clinical trial enrollment.[12]

---

[a] Division of Cardiology, St. Michael's Hospital, 30 Bond Street, Toronto, Ontario M5B 1W8, Canada; [b] Waikato Hospital, 183 Pembroke Street, Hamilton 3204, New Zealand
* Corresponding author.
E-mail address: neil.fam@unityhealth.to
Twitter: @DanielHagemeyer (D.H.)

Intervent Cardiol Clin 11 (2022) 103–112
https://doi.org/10.1016/j.iccl.2021.09.006
2211-7458/22/© 2021 Elsevier Inc. All rights reserved.

Owing to the complex and variable anatomy of the tricuspid valve, imaging plays a crucial role in most transcatheter procedures, and advanced imaging tools are required.[13] Transesophageal echocardiography (TEE) is considered to be the gold standard. However, several technical issues are faced when it comes to tricuspid valve imaging, for example, the anterior location of the valve and therefore longer distance between the esophagus and the right side of the heart, right heart enlargement, as well as adverse acoustic shadowing from cardiac prostheses, the interatrial septum, or the device delivery system. In a study looking at image quality in 211 patients, TEE optimally visualized the tricuspid valve in only 11% of patients, whereas the visualization of the mitral valve was optimal in 85% to 91%.[14] In clinical practice, some patients may have contraindications to the use of TEE (Table 1). Intracardiac echocardiography (ICE) can overcome many of these issues and therefore plays an emerging role for intraprocedural guidance. In this review, we discuss the inherent strengths and challenges of TEE and ICE in tricuspid valve interventions.

BACKGROUND: INTRACARDIAC ECHOCARDIOGRAPHY FOR STRUCTURAL HEART INTERVENTIONS

Transvenous ICE was already used in 1981 but did not find its way into routine clinical practice for a long time.[16] In 1991, Valdes-Cruz and colleagues[17] reported its first successful use in structural heart disease for percutaneous atrial septal defect closure in piglets. In the beginning, ICE was mainly used to guide atrial septal defect closures and transseptal puncture in electrophysiological procedures. With further development of the probes and the introduction of steerable phased-array devices, the range of applications expanded.

Although to date TEE is still most commonly used for procedural guidance, there has been a growing interest in intracardiac imaging for various kinds of structural heart interventions under conscious sedation for a less invasive approach.

Existing data demonstrate that ICE can be safely used for guiding ablation of cardiac arrhythmias, atrial septal defect closure, left atrial appendage closure, as well as percutaneous pulmonary valve replacement.[18–25] Indeed, in 2014, 50% of all interatrial communication closures were ICE guided.[26] ICE was used in 67% of atrial fibrillation ablations and was associated with a lower risk of repeat ablation but with a slightly higher risk of bleeding.[27] Also, valve interventions including percutaneous balloon mitral valve valvuloplasty were successfully guided with ICE only.[28–30] In a single-center study, ICE was used as an additional imaging tool to fluoroscopy to minimize contrast volume in transcatheter aortic valve replacement.[31] The procedure that is most similar to transcatheter tricuspid valve repair (TTVr) is percutaneous mitral valve repair with the MitraClip (Abbott Vascular). ICE was used in a small number of cases, mainly in addition to TEE when imaging was suboptimal.[32–35]

The use of ICE for visualizing the RV and the tricuspid valve was comprehensively described by Ren and colleagues.[36,37] In a case report, the use of ICE to guide transcatheter tricuspid valve-in-valve implantation was described.[38] Robinson and colleagues[39] reported the use of an S8-3T MicroTEE echocardiography probe (Philips, Amsterdam, The Netherlands) in a sterile sleeve, which was advanced to the right atrium via the right internal jugular vein. With this approach, they were able to provide multiplanar echocardiographic images to guide percutaneous tricuspid repair.[39]

Several studies have conducted head-to-head comparisons of ICE and TEE in various structural heart interventions. A single-center cohort study

Table 1	
Contraindications to transesophageal echocardiography as suggested by Hilberath et al	
Absolute Contraindications to TEE	**Relative Contraindications to TEE**
Perforated viscous	Atlantoaxial joint disease with restricted cervical mobility
Esophageal pathology (stricture, trauma, tumor, scleroderma, Mallory-Weiss tear, diverticulum, varices)	Prior radiation to the chest
Active upper GI bleeding	Symptomatic hiatal hernia
Recent upper GI surgery	History of GI surgery
Esophagectomy, esophagogastrectomy	Recent upper GI bleeding
	Esophagitis, peptic ulcer disease
	Thoracoabdominal aneurysm
	Barrett's esophagus
	History of dysphagia
	Coagulopathy, thrombocytopenia

Abbreviation: GI, gastrointestinal.

compared the efficacy and safety of ICE in the left atrium under local anesthesia (n = 109) with TEE under general anesthesia (n = 107) for procedural guidance for transcatheter left atrial appendage occlusion. Technical success was achieved in 99% of both the TEE and ICE group. Major periprocedural complications occurred in 4.7% of the TEE group and 1.8% of the ICE group. Contrast usage and total time in the catheterization laboratory were significantly lower in the ICE group.[40]

Even though TEE is considered a safe procedure, the risk of TEE-related injuries is underappreciated. In a prospective study of 50 patients undergoing TEE-guided structural cardiac interventions (mitral and tricuspid valve repair, left atrial appendage closure, and paravalvular leak closure), an esophagogastroduodenoscopy was performed before and immediately after the procedure. The postprocedural esophagogastroduodenoscopy showed a new injury in 86% (n = 43/50) of the patients, with complex lesions (intramural hematoma, mucosal laceration) accounting for 40% (n = 20 of 50) of the cases. Independent factors associated with an increased risk of complex lesions were a longer procedural time and a suboptimal image quality.[41] Both factors play a crucial role in tricuspid valve interventions.

INTRACARDIAC ECHOCARDIOGRAPHY FOR TRICUSPID INTERVENTIONS

In tricuspid valve edge-to-edge repair, imaging is essential for device steering, clip positioning, leaflet grasping, and confirmation of insertion. ICE was already reported in the early era of TTVr in 2016. Hammerstingl and colleagues[42] reported the first cases of TTVr with the MitraClip system, and ICE was used as an adjunct to TEE for procedural guidance. One year later, a case report described a patient with previous esophagectomy treated with TTVr guided with ICE and fluoroscopy alone.[43] Similarly, a patient with significant shadowing of the tricuspid valve leaflets by a mitral annuloplasty ring underwent successful TTVr using ICE guidance (Fig. 1).[44] Latib and colleagues[45] described a case of percutaneous tricuspid valve annuloplasty in a patient with a large esophageal diverticulum only guided by TTE, multi slice CT, and ICE. Lane and colleagues[46] reported a case of TTVr with the MitraClip system where imaging was challenging due to shadowing from a tricuspid annuloplasty band, and grasping could only be visualized with ICE. Although ICE can play an important role in procedural imaging for percutaneous tricuspid valve repair, it is generally

reserved as an adjunct to TEE given the cost and the current lack of real-time multiplanar imaging technology.[47]

Curio and colleagues[48] compared procedural safety and outcomes up to 30 days after tricuspid interventions between ICE/TEE and TEE alone. The investigators found that 50% of the patients had insufficient visualization of the tricuspid valve with TEE only. Yet, in two-thirds of the patients in this group, clip implantation was possible by using ICE, highlighting the role of ICE to facilitate intervention. The safety end point was the same in both groups (0% procedural complications).[48]

4D volume ICE has the potential to revolutionize tricuspid intervention and is undergoing continuous technological improvement. Davidson and colleagues[49] reported the systematic use of 4D volume ICE (Siemens Healthineers, Erlangen, Germany) as an intraprocedural imaging modality in 26 patients undergoing Cardioband implantation. The investigators stated that visualization, especially of the lateral annulus, improved compared with TEE.[49] In our institution, we used 4D volume ICE for transcatheter tricuspid valve replacement with the EVOQUE system (Edwards Lifesciences) in a patient with torrential TR (Fig. 2).

Various approaches for guiding tricuspid valve procedures have been described, but ICE imaging planes are not standardized.[44,48,50,51] Partially, this is due to the complex and variable anatomy of the tricuspid valve, which requires individual adaptations. In the following, we describe the basic views that can be obtained in most patients. In the "home view" the probe faces anteriorly without any flex. In this position, the right atrium, the RV, and the tricuspid valve can be visualized. By flexing anteriorly and toward the right atrial free wall (left/right knob) with subtle clock/counterclockwise catheter rotation, the clip arms and their position can be assessed in relation to the leaflets. Usually, this is considered to be an acceptable orthogonal long-axis grasping view. Optimizing the view of anteroseptal commissure can be done by advancing the catheter higher in the RA, whereas the posteroseptal commissure can be visualized by retracting the catheter. Only small movements are necessary to optimize the view, and it is helpful to have a second operator to maintain the view during the intervention.

ACCESS, CONTRAINDICATIONS, AND COMPLICATIONS

After obtaining venous access in the left femoral vein, preclosure with Perclose ProGlide System

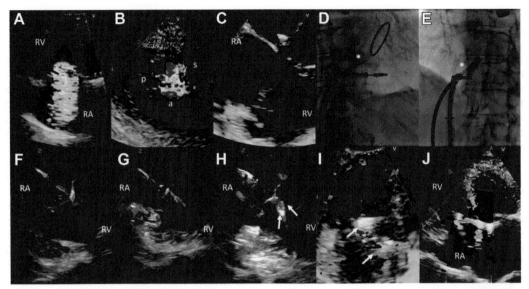

Fig. 1. Intracardiac echocardiography for guidance of transcatheter tricuspid repair. (*A*) Baseline TTE RV-focused view with color Doppler demonstrating torrential TR. (*B*) Baseline TEE transgastric view of tricuspid valve demonstrating torrential TR. (*C*) Intraprocedural TEE demonstrating shadowing of tricuspid valve leaflets by a mitral annuloplasty ring. (*D*) Fluoroscopy in right anterior oblique projection of ICE catheter position (*asterisk* indicates ICE catheter). (*E*) Fluoroscopy in LAO projection of ICE catheter position (*asterisk* indicates ICE catheter). (*F*) Intraprocedural ICE view of MitraClip grasping of tricuspid valve posterior and septal leaflets. (*G*) Intraprocedural ICE view of first MitraClip demonstrating tissue bridge. (*H*) Intraprocedural ICE view following deployment of 2 MitraClips (*arrows* indicates clips). (*I*) Intraprocedural TEE transgastric view of tricuspid valve with simultaneous color Doppler after implantation of 2 MitraClips (*arrows* indicates clips). (*J*) Postprocedural TTE apical 4-chamber view demonstrating sustained TR reduction at 1-month follow-up. a, anterior; p, posterior; RA, right atrium; s, septal; TTE, transthoracic echocardiography.

(Abbott Vascular) can be used to facilitate post-procedural vessel hemostasis. After insertion of a long 10F sheath into the inferior vena cava, the ICE probe is advanced into the midright atrium under fluoroscopic guidance. There are not many contraindications for the use of ICE; its use is mainly limited to inadequate vascular access. Other contraindicated conditions include the presence of an intracardiac thrombus, sepsis, major coagulation abnormalities, IVC occlusion, and deep vein thrombosis. Until today reliable systematic data about complication rate related to intracardiac imaging is missing. The possible complications are the same as the ones occurring during right heart catheterization; especially, one should be aware of any vascular complications during catheter advancement because it is not wire guided. Also, to identify bleeding complications, the incision site should be inspected regularly. Furthermore, cardiac arrhythmias can occur when the probe interacts with the RV wall. Moreover, the risk of thrombus formation is lesser on the venous side, but adequate anticoagulation should be administered. Last, cardiac tamponade and infection at the incision site are very rare.

INTRACARDIAC ECHOCARDIOGRAPHY DEVICES

The technical details of the most commonly used intracardiac ultrasound probes are summarized in this section. All probes are designed to be single use, but the 2D probes may be commercially resterilized. The ViewFlex Xtra (Abbott Vascular) is a 9F steerable ICE probe with a working length of 90 cm. The visualization angle is up to 90°, and an integrated connector eliminates the need for a sterile sleeve. This probe has a penetration depth of 18 cm and a deflection angle of 120°. The device can generate 2D, continuous wave doppler, pulse wave doppler, color Doppler, and M-mode.

The AcuNav (Siemens Healthineers) is a comparable system; it comes as a 90-cm 10F catheter, which has 4-way steering in 2 planes (160° in each direction). The imaging modes are 2D, harmonics, M-mode, CW, PW, color Doppler, and tissue tracking.

For ICE to serve as the sole procedural imaging tool and to avoid TEE with general anesthesia, multiplanar, real-time 4D ICE is needed. With progressive technological improvements,

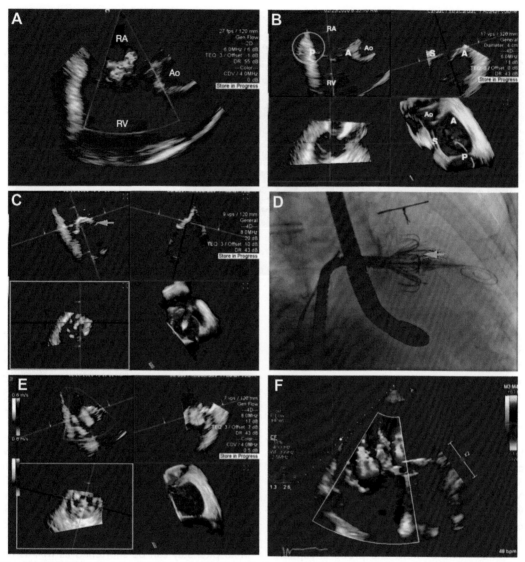

Fig. 2. (A) 2D ICE with color Doppler. (B) 4D ICE multi planar reconstruction (MPR). (C, D) 4D ICE MPR and fluoroscopy of EVOQUE valve. (E) 4D ICE MPR color Doppler. (F) Transthoracic echocardiography with color Doppler at follow-up. RA, right atrium; Ao, aorta; P, posterior; A, anterior; S, septal.

4D ICE has emerged and will soon be ready for "prime time." At present, there is only one commercially available 4D ICE probe (Siemens), with two about to enter the market (NuVera and Philips).

The ACUSON AcuNav V catheter (Siemens Healthineers) is a 12F 3D volumetric ICE system; it is capable of volumetric reconstruction of intracardiac images with real-time 3D formatting (volume size of $22° \times 90°$) (**Fig. 3**). The feasibility to guide percutaneous transcatheter therapy (closure of the patent foramen ovale or atrial septal defects, and balloon valvuloplasty for mitral stenosis) was shown.[52–54] The catheter

was also successfully used for percutaneous mitral valve edge-to-edge repair.[55]

In addition, this system was shown to be feasible for guidance of TTVr with the MitraClip system in 5 cases at 2 institutions.[56] The product just received CE mark in June 2021.

The NuVision (Nuvera, Los Gatos CA, USA; recently acquired by Biosense Webster, USA) is a 4D ICE probe with a 10F steerable shaft, a $90° \times 90°$ field of view, and greater than 15 cm ultrasound penetration depth. At TCT 2020, Ebner and Latib presented the first-in-human experience with this new device for structural heart procedures[57]; it was a prospective,

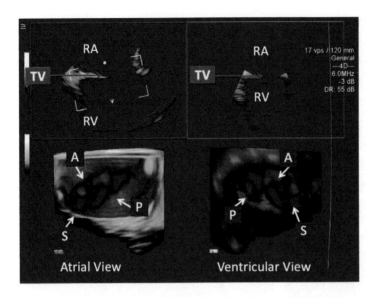

Fig. 3. ICE of the tricuspid valve with Acuson AcuNav Volume ICE catheter (with permission of Siemens Healthineers). RA, right atrium; TV, tricuspid valve; a, anterior; p, posterior; s, septal.

nonrandomized, single-center feasibility study of 5 subjects. In this very small study, all primary performance end points were met in all patients and no adverse events were reported. The image quality and catheter performance were rated as very good (5 on a Likert scale) in greater than 98%.

In July 2021, Philips reported the first structural heart procedure (left atrial appendage closure) using the new VeriSight Pro real-time 3D ICE catheter (Philips, Amsterdam, The Netherlands) at Mayo Clinic. The device has a 9F steerable shaft, and a minimum sheath size of 10F is required; it has a useable length of 90 cm with a deflection range of 120° and 90° × 90° field of view. The probe is capable of x-plane and live 3D volume and color-flow imaging. The probe is now available on a limited basis in the United States.

INTRACARDIAC ECHOCARDIOGRAPHY: PROS AND CONS

For ICE, additional access at the contralateral side is usually obtained with a 10F sheath. The additional access may lead to complications like hematoma, arteriovenous fistula, and patient discomfort, which can be partly prevented by using ultrasound-guided puncture and sufficient local anesthesia.

Once the ultrasound probe is positioned in the right atrium and an adequate image of the tricuspid valve is achieved, it can be challenging to maintain a stable view of the intracardiac structures. Having a dedicated team member to operate the probe can overcome this problem. As with any other device, ICE has a learning curve until the probe manipulation can be mastered in a way that clear and reliable images are achieved. Owing to increasing cost pressures, many decisions in the health care system are driven by financial considerations. Therefore, the extra costs for an intracardiac ultrasound catheter must be well justified. The upfront costs of the single-use catheters are high but can be mitigated by commercial probe resterilization. If ICE is used as a substitute for TEE, the costs of the anesthesiologist and assistants as well as the anesthetic drugs and equipment can be saved. By avoiding general anesthesia, the duration of in-hospital stay can be shortened as well as the case duration, because the time of induction and recovery from the anesthesia is removed.[18,19]

By avoiding general anesthesia, the patient is less exposed to common risks such as aspiration, postoperative nausea and vomiting, airway irritation, or damage of the teeth because of intubation. Because the population requiring tricuspid valve intervention has an advanced age and often takes multiple medications, the risk for adverse drug effects is higher.

Another aspect of general anesthesia is the influence on the hemodynamics by lowering the systemic blood pressure and, due to mechanical ventilation, the increase the intrathoracic pressure; this can change the severity of TR and make the evaluation of procedural success challenging. By using ICE in an awake patient, assessment of TR reduction is more realistic.

Table 2
Disadvantages and advantages of intracardiac echocardiography

Advantages of ICE	Disadvantages of ICE
• No acoustic shadowing from other intracardiac devices • No acoustic shadowing of the clip delivery system • Alternative if TEE is contraindicated • Shorter procedure times and with faster turnaround • No general anesthesia needed • Hemodynamics not influenced by anesthetic drugs and mechanical ventilation	• Second venous access needed • Instability of probe during intervention • Additional cost of the ultrasound catheter • Learning curve

Because staff costs are usually a large part of the overall costs, an interventional cardiologist may also perform the ICE imaging; this saves the cost of an additional echocardiographer and TEE equipment. Alboliras and Hijazi compared the costs for percutaneous device closure of atrial septal defects in children and adults using the Amplatzer Septal Occluder using TEE only with using ICE only. The costs were similar when using ICE and TEE (US$ 33,563 vs US$ 32,812, P = .42), even though there incurred additional expenses due to the ICE interpretation by the echocardiographer (depending on the expertise of the interventionalist this may be omitted).[58]

Another aspect that is especially of importance during the coronavirus disease 2019 pandemic is the fact that all aerosol-generating procedures, which have an increased risk of transmission of respiratory virus (such as TEE), should be avoided or require special personal protective equipment (Table 2).[59]

SUMMARY

Although TEE is currently the gold standard imaging modality for structural heart interventions, ICE plays an emerging role especially in guiding percutaneous valve procedures, either as an adjunctive imaging tool when TEE cannot provide sufficient images or as a substitute in patients in whom TEE is contraindicated. ICE

negates the need for general anesthesia with its associated risks, which is particularly appealing in the elderly or clinically tenuous patient. In the future, 4D ICE with wider acquisition volumes and real-time MPR has the potential to replace TEE for procedural guidance with advances in imaging technology.

CLINICS CARE POINTS

ICE

• can be of use when transesophageal echo views are limited
• can be used as an alternative to TEE
• is likely to shorten the procedural time
• has been shown to be a safe procedure
• requires a learning curve.

DISCLOSURE

N.P. Fam is a consultant for Edwards Lifesciences and Abbott. Daniel Hagemeyer is supported by Gottfried Und Julia Bangerter-Rhyner-Stiftung, Bern. The remaining authors have no disclosures.

REFERENCES

1. Singh JP, Evans JC, Levy D, et al. Prevalence and clinical determinants of mitral, tricuspid, and aortic regurgitation (The Framingham Heart Study). Am J Cardiol 1999;83(6):897–902.
2. Nath J, Foster E, Heidenreich PA. Impact of tricuspid regurgitation on long-term survival. J Am Coll Cardiol 2004;43(3):405–9.
3. Chorin E, Rozenbaum Z, Topilsky Y, et al. Tricuspid regurgitation and long-term clinical outcomes. Eur Heart J Cardiovasc Imaging 2020;21(2):157–65.
4. Zack CJ, Fender EA, Chandrashekar P, et al. National trends and outcomes in isolated tricuspid valve surgery. J Am Coll Cardiol 2017;70(24):2953–60.
5. Topilsky Y, Khanna AD, Oh JK, et al. Preoperative factors associated with adverse outcome after tricuspid valve replacement. Circulation 2011;123(18):1929–39.
6. Taramasso M, Hahn RT, Alessandrini H, et al. The International Multicenter TriValve Registry: which patients are undergoing transcatheter tricuspid repair? JACC Cardiovasc Interv 2017;10(19):1982–90.
7. Kodali S, Hahn RT, Eleid MF, et al. Feasibility study of the transcatheter valve repair system for severe

tricuspid regurgitation. J Am Coll Cardiol 2021; 77(4):345–56.

8. Mehr M, Taramasso M, Besler C, et al. 1-year outcomes after edge-to-edge valve repair for symptomatic tricuspid regurgitation: results from the TriValve registry. JACC Cardiovasc Interv 2019; 12(15):1451–61.

9. Lurz P, Stephan von Bardeleben R, Weber M, et al. Transcatheter edge-to-edge repair for treatment of tricuspid regurgitation. J Am Coll Cardiol 2021; 77(3):229–39.

10. Nickenig G, Weber M, Schueler R, et al. 6-month outcomes of tricuspid valve reconstruction for patients with severe tricuspid regurgitation. J Am Coll Cardiol 2019;73(15):1905–15.

11. Davidson CJ, Lim DS, Smith RL, et al. Early feasibility study of cardioband tricuspid system for functional tricuspid regurgitation: 30-day outcomes. JACC Cardiovasc Interv 2021;14(1):41–50.

12. Fam NP, von Bardeleben RS, Hensey M, et al. Transfemoral Transcatheter tricuspid valve replacement with the EVOQUE system: a multicenter, observational, first-in-human experience. JACC Cardiovasc Interv 2021;14(5):501–11.

13. Dahou A, Levin D, Reisman M, et al. Anatomy and physiology of the tricuspid valve. JACC Cardiovasc Imaging 2019;12(3):458–68.

14. Sugeng L, Shernan SK, Salgo IS, et al. Live 3-Dimensional transesophageal echocardiography. initial experience using the fully-sampled matrix array probe. J Am Coll Cardiol 2008;52(6):446–9.

15. Hilberath JN, Oakes DA, Shernan SK, et al. Safety of transesophageal echocardiography. J Am Soc Echocardiogr 2010;23(11):1115–27.

16. Glassman E, Kronzon I. Transvenous intracardiac echocardiography. Am J Cardiol 1981;47(6): 1255–9.

17. Valdes-Cruz LM, Sideris E, Sahn DJ, et al. Transvascular intracardiac applications of a miniaturized phased-array ultrasonic endoscope. Initial experience with intracardiac imaging in piglets. Circulation 1991;83(3):1023–7.

18. Boccalandro F, Baptista E, Muench A, et al. Comparison of intracardiac echocardiography versus transesophageal echocardiography guidance for percutaneous transcatheter closure of atrial septal defect. Am J Cardiol 2004;93(4): 437–40.

19. Bartel T, Konorza T, Neudorf U, et al. Intracardiac echocardiography: An ideal guiding tool for device closure of interatrial communications. Eur J Echocardiogr 2005;6(2):92–6.

20. Marrouche NF, Martin DO, Wazni O, et al. Phased-array intracardiac echocardiography monitoring during pulmonary vein isolation in patients with atrial fibrillation impact on outcome and complications. Circulation 2003;107(21):2710–6.

21. Awad SM, Masood SA, Gonzalez I, et al. The use of intracardiac echocardiography during percutaneous pulmonary valve replacement. Pediatr Cardiol 2015;36(1):76–83.

22. Bartel T, Konorza T, Arjumand J, et al. Intracardiac echocardiography is superior to conventional monitoring for guiding device closure of interatrial communications. Circulation 2003;107(6):795–7.

23. Rigatelli G, Pedon L, Zecchel R, et al. Long-term outcomes and complications of intracardiac echocardiography-assisted patent foramen ovale closure in 1,000 consecutive patients; long-term outcomes and complications of intracardiac echocardiography-assisted patent foramen ovale closure in 1,000 consecutive patients. J Interv Cardiol 2016;29(5):530–8.

24. Ponnuthurai FA, van Gaal WJ, Burchell A, et al. Safety and feasibility of day case patent foramen ovale (PFO) closure facilitated by intracardiac echocardiography. Int J Cardiol 2009;131(3):438–40.

25. Reddy VY, Gibson DN, Kar S, et al. Post-approval U.S. experience with left atrial appendage closure for stroke prevention in atrial fibrillation. J Am Coll Cardiol 2017;69(3):253–61.

26. Alqahtani F, Bhirud A, Aljohani S, et al. Intracardiac versus transesophageal echocardiography to guide transcatheter closure of interatrial communications: Nationwide trend and comparative analysis. J Interv Cardiol 2017;30(3):234–41.

27. Steinberg BA, Hammill BG, Daubert JP, et al. Periprocedural imaging and outcomes after catheter ablation of atrial fibrillation. Heart 2014;100(23): 1871–7.

28. Salem MI, Makaryus AN, Kort S, et al. Intracardiac echocardiography using the AcuNav ultrasound catheter during percutaneous balloon mitral valvuloplasty. J Am Soc Echocardiogr 2002;15(12):1533–7.

29. Green NE, Hansgen AR, Carroll JD. Initial clinical experience with intracardiac echocardiography in guiding balloon mitral valvuloplasty: technique, safety, utility, and limitations. Catheter Cardiovasc Interv 2004;63(3):385–94.

30. Saji M, Ragosta M, Dent J, et al. Use of intracardiac echocardiography to guide percutaneous transluminal mitral commissurotomy: a 20-patient case series. Catheter Cardiovasc Interv 2016;87(2):E69–74.

31. Bartel T, Bonaros N, Edlinger M, et al. Intracardiac echo and reduced radiocontrast requirements during TAVR. JACC Cardiovasc Imaging 2014;7(3): 319–20.

32. Henning A, Mueller II, Mueller K, et al. Percutaneous edge-to-edge mitral valve repair escorted

by left atrial intracardiac echocardiography (ICE). Circulation 2014;130(20):e173–4.

33. Saji M, Rossi AM, Ailawadi G, et al. Adjunctive intracardiac echocardiography imaging from the left ventricle to guide percutaneous mitral valve repair with the mitraclip in patients with failed prior surgical rings. Catheter Cardiovasc Interv 2016;87(2): E75–82.

34. Yap J, Rogers JH, Aman E, et al. MitraClip implantation guided by volumetric intracardiac echocardiography: technique and feasibility in patients intolerant to transesophageal echocardiography. Cardiovasc Revasc Med 2021;28S:85–8.

35. Alkhouli M, Eleid MF, Michellena H, et al. Complementary roles of intracardiac and transoesophageal echocardiography in transcatheter tricuspid interventions. EuroIntervention 2020;15(17):1514–5.

36. Ren JF, Callans DJ, Marchlinski FE. Tricuspid regurgitation severity associated with positioning of RV lead or other etiology assessed by intracardiac echocardiography. JACC Cardiovasc Imaging 2014;7(12):1285–6.

37. Ren JF, Callans DJ, Marchlinski FE. A simplified quantitative evaluation of right ventricular anatomy and function by intracardiac echocardiography. JACC Heart Fail 2014;2(2):198–9.

38. Saji M, Ailawadi G, Izarnotegui V, et al. Intracardiac echocardiography during transcatheter tricuspid valve-in-valve implantation. Cardiovasc Interv Ther 2018;33(3):285–7.

39. Robinson AA, Chadwell K, Fowler DE, et al. Multiplane intracardiac echocardiography: a novel system to guide percutaneous tricuspid repair. JACC Cardiovasc Interventions 2018;11(24):2540–2.

40. Korsholm K, Jensen JM, Nielsen-Kudsk JE. Intracardiac echocardiography from the left atrium for procedural guidance of transcatheter left atrial appendage occlusion. JACC Cardiovasc Interventions 2017;10(21):2198–206.

41. Freitas-Ferraz AB, Bernier M, Vaillancourt R, et al. Safety of transesophageal echocardiography to guide structural cardiac interventions. J Am Coll Cardiol 2020;75(25):3164–73.

42. Hammerstingl C, Schueler R, Malasa M, et al. Transcatheter treatment of severe tricuspid regurgitation with the MitraClip system. Eur Heart J 2016;37(10): 849–53.

43. Pozzoli A, Taramasso M, Zuber M, et al. Transcatheter tricuspid valve repair with the MitraClip system using intracardiac echocardiography: proof of concept. EuroIntervention 2017;13(12):e1452–3.

44. Fam NP, Samargandy S, Gandhi S, et al. Intracardiac echocardiography for guidance of transcatheter tricuspid edge-to-edge repair. EuroIntervention 2018;14(9):e1004–5.

45. Latib A, Mangieri A, Vicentini L, et al. Percutaneous tricuspid valve annuloplasty under conscious sedation (with only fluoroscopic and intracardiac echocardiography monitoring). JACC Cardiovasc Interv 2017;10(6):620–1.

46. Lane CE, Thaden JJ, Eleid MF, et al. The dynamic duo - intracardiac and transesophageal echocardiography in transcatheter edge-to-edge tricuspid valve repair. JACC Cardiovasc Interv 2021;14(11): e125–6.

47. Ancona F, Stella S, Taramasso M, et al. Multimodality imaging of the tricuspid valve with implication for percutaneous repair approaches. Heart 2017; 103(14):1073–81.

48. Curio J, Abulgasim K, Kasner M, et al. Intracardiac echocardiography to enable successful edge-to-edge transcatheter tricuspid valve repair in patients with insufficient TEE quality. Clin Hemorheol Microcirc 2020;76(2):199–210.

49. Davidson CJ, Abramson S, Smith RL, et al. Transcatheter Tricuspid Repair With the Use of 4-Dimensional Intracardiac Echocardiography. JACC Cardiovasc Imaging 2021;1–6. https://doi.org/10.1016/j.jcmg.2021.01.029.

50. Asrress KN, Mitchell ARJ. Intracardiac echocardiography. Heart 2009;95(4):327–31.

51. Alkhouli M, Hijazi ZM, Holmes DR, et al. Intracardiac Echocardiography in Structural Heart Disease Interventions. JACC Cardiovasc Interventions 2018;11(21):2133–47.

52. Silvestry FE, Kadakia MB, Willhide J, et al. Initial experience with a novel real-time three-dimensional intracardiac ultrasound system to guide percutaneous cardiac structural interventions: a phase 1 feasibility study of volume intracardiac echocardiography in the assessment of patients with structural heart disease undergoing percutaneous transcatheter therapy. J Am Soc Echocardiogr 2014;27(9):978–83.

53. Fontes-Carvalho R, Sampaio F, Ribeiro J, et al. Three-dimensional intracardiac echocardiography: A new promising imaging modality to potentially guide cardiovascular interventions. Eur Heart J Cardiovasc Imaging 2013;14(10):1028.

54. Cunnington C, Hampshaw SA, Mahadevan VS. Utility of real-time three-dimensional intracardiac echocardiography for patent foramen ovale closure. Heart 2013;99(23):1789–90.

55. Patzelt J, Schreieck J, Camus E, et al. Percutaneous mitral valve edge-to-edge repair using volume intracardiac echocardiography—first in human experience. CASE (Phila) 2017;1(1):41–3.

56. Tang GHL, Yakubov SJ, Sanchez Soto CE. 4-Dimensional intracardiac echocardiography in transcatheter tricuspid valve repair with the MitraClip system. JACC Cardiovasc Imaging 2020;13(7): 1591–600.

57. Ebner A, Latib A. First in human experience (FIH) with novel real time 3d intracardiac

echocardiography (4D ICE) catheter a virtually supported clinical study performed during global pandemic. In: TCT Connect. 2020.

58. Alboliras ET, Hijazi ZM. Comparison of costs of intracardiac echocardiography and transesophageal echocardiography in monitoring percutaneous device closure of atrial septal defect in children and adults. Am J Cardiol 2004;94(5):690–2.

59. Hung J, Abraham TP, Cohen MS, et al. ASE Statement on the Reintroduction of Echocardiographic Services during the COVID-19 Pandemic. J Am Soc Echocardiogr 2020;33(8):1034–9.

Moving?

Make sure your subscription moves with you!

To notify us of your new address, find your **Clinics Account Number** (located on your mailing label above your name), and contact customer service at:

Email: journalscustomerservice-usa@elsevier.com

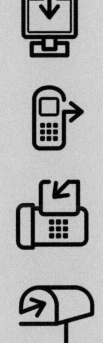

800-654-2452 (subscribers in the U.S. & Canada)
314-447-8871 (subscribers outside of the U.S. & Canada)

Fax number: 314-447-8029

Elsevier Health Sciences Division
Subscription Customer Service
3251 Riverport Lane
Maryland Heights, MO 63043

*To ensure uninterrupted delivery of your subscription, please notify us at least 4 weeks in advance of move.

Printed and bound by CPI Group (UK) Ltd, Croydon, CR0 4YY

03/10/2024

01040363-0006